IN-DEMAND CAREERS

# BE A PHYSICIAN ASSISTANT

by Amy C. Rea

BrightPoint Press

San Diego, CA

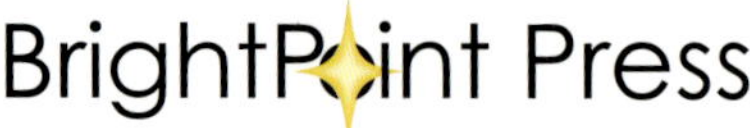


an imprint of ReferencePoint Press, Inc.
Printed in the United States

For more information, contact:
BrightPoint Press
PO Box 27779
San Diego, CA 92198
www.BrightPointPress.com



LIBRARY OF CONGRESS CATALOGING-IN-PUBLICATION DATA

Name: Rea, Amy C., author.
Title: Be a physician assistant / by Amy C. Rea.
Description: San Diego, CA: ReferencePoint Press, 2026 | Series: In-demand careers | Audience: Grade 7 to 9 | Includes bibliographical references and index.
Identifiers: ISBN: 9781678211226 (hardcover) | ISBN: 9781678211233 (eBook)
The complete Library of Congress record is available at www.loc.gov.

# CONTENTS

# AT A GLANCE

- A physician assistant (PA) is a health care professional who can diagnose and treat patients.
- PAs can do medical procedures such as stitching up wounds. They also teach patients about healthy living.
- Some PAs work in primary care. Other PAs specialize in cardiology or surgery.
- PAs can work in clinics, hospitals, nursing homes, military bases, or schools.
- A PA needs an undergraduate degree followed by a postgraduate degree. Both degree programs vary in length.
- A PA must become certified and earn a license in their state to practice medicine.

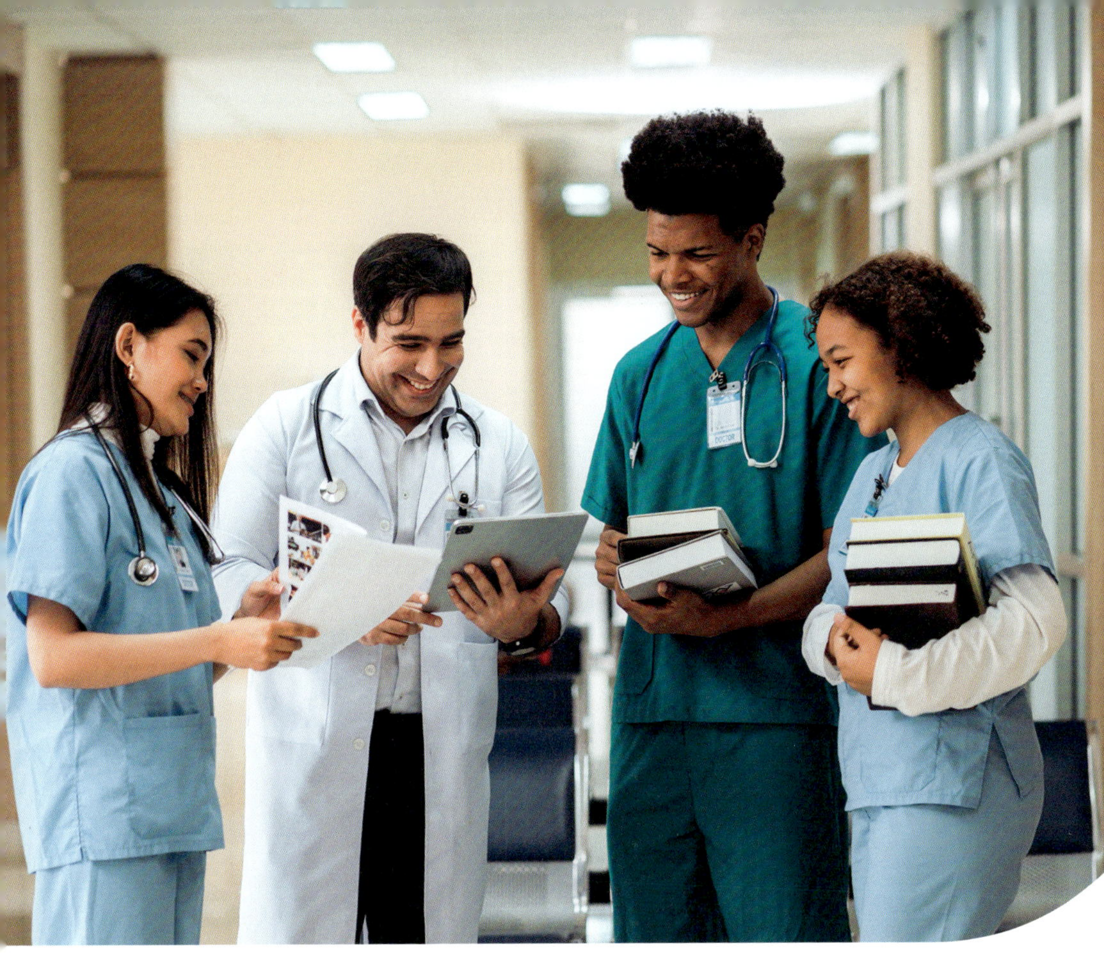

- Part of a PA's education is clinical rotations. PAs get to meet and work with patients.
- Some PAs work Monday through Friday during the day. Others may work nights, weekends, and holidays.
- Due to a shortage of doctors, there will be a greater demand for PAs in the next 10 years.

# MANY PATIENTS, MANY MEDICAL TASKS

It is another busy morning. Physician assistant (PA) Joseph Carter works at a health clinic in Santa Ynez, California. He starts his day by reviewing lab work. Carter also calls his patients. He lets them know their test results.

Then, Carter sees patients. His first patient has a bad cough. Carter diagnoses the patient with a viral infection. It is affecting the patient's airways and lungs.

**Physician assistants make sure patients understand their test results.**

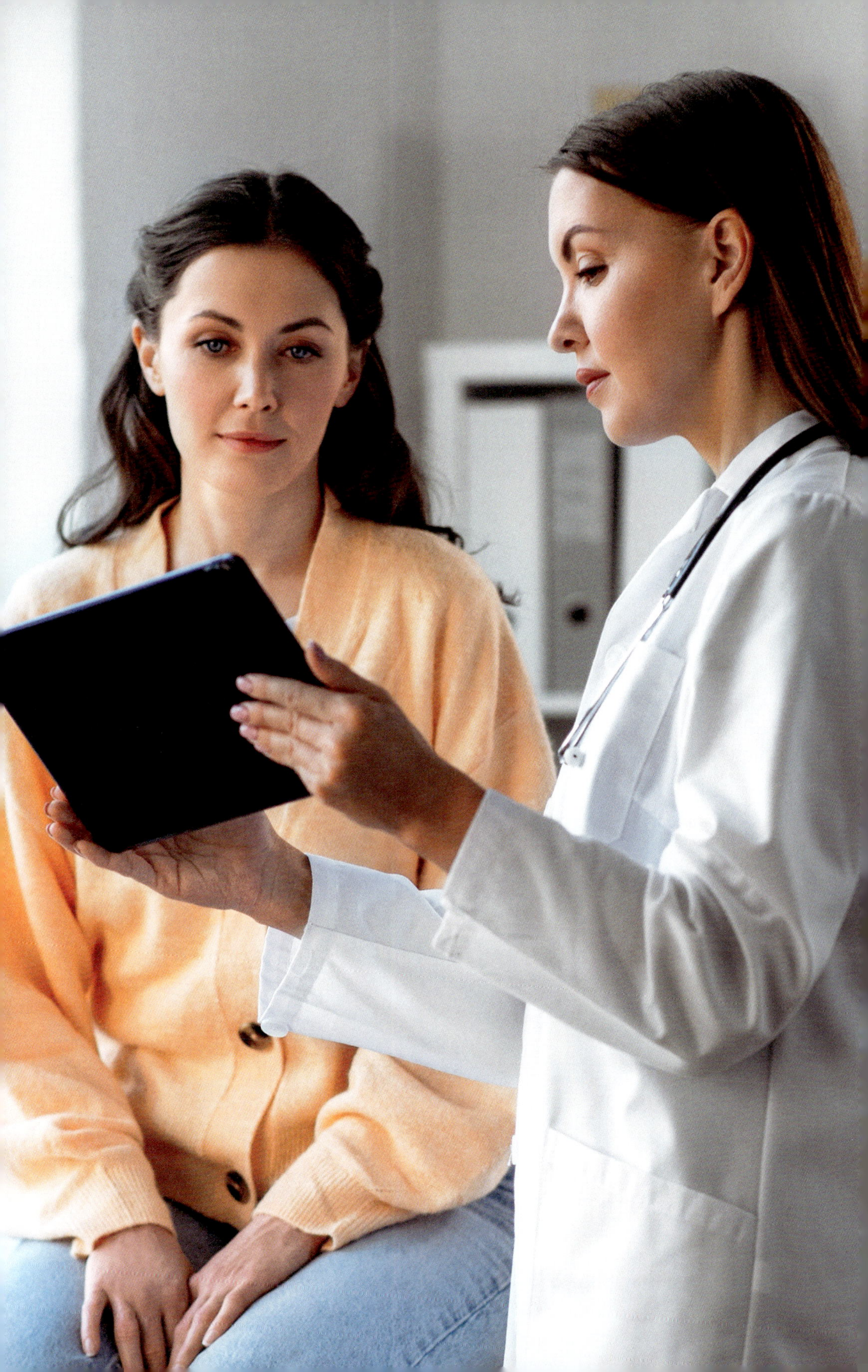

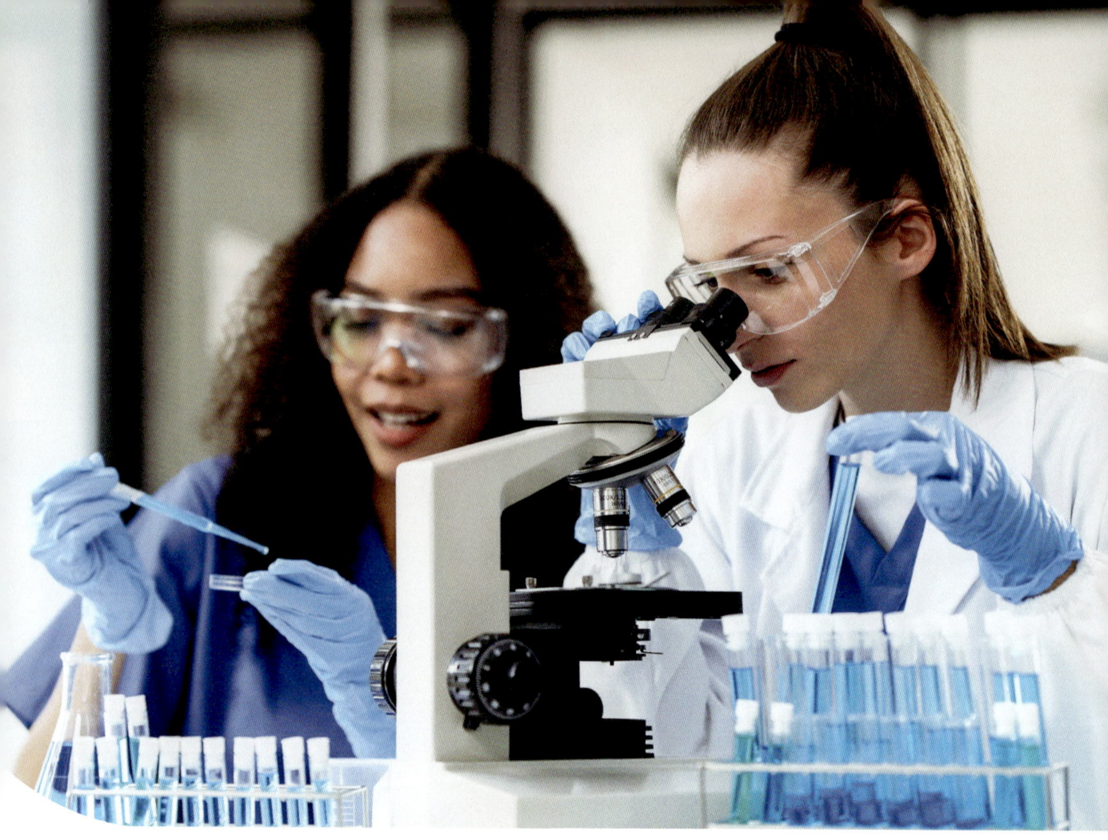

**Lab tests may require samples of a patient's body fluids. These include blood or urine.**

His next patient has **diabetes**. Carter reviews the patient's health care plan. The plan describes what the patient needs for treatment. He then prescribes medication. He also orders lab tests.

Carter sees between fifteen and twenty patients each day. They may include someone who needs stitches for a bad cut on a finger. Another may be a child who has a fever. Carter updates patient records after examining each patient.

Carter's favorite part of his job is getting to meet with his patients. He sometimes interacts with the same patients over the years. He gets to be a part of their daily

**PAs learn to listen to and build positive relationships with patients.**

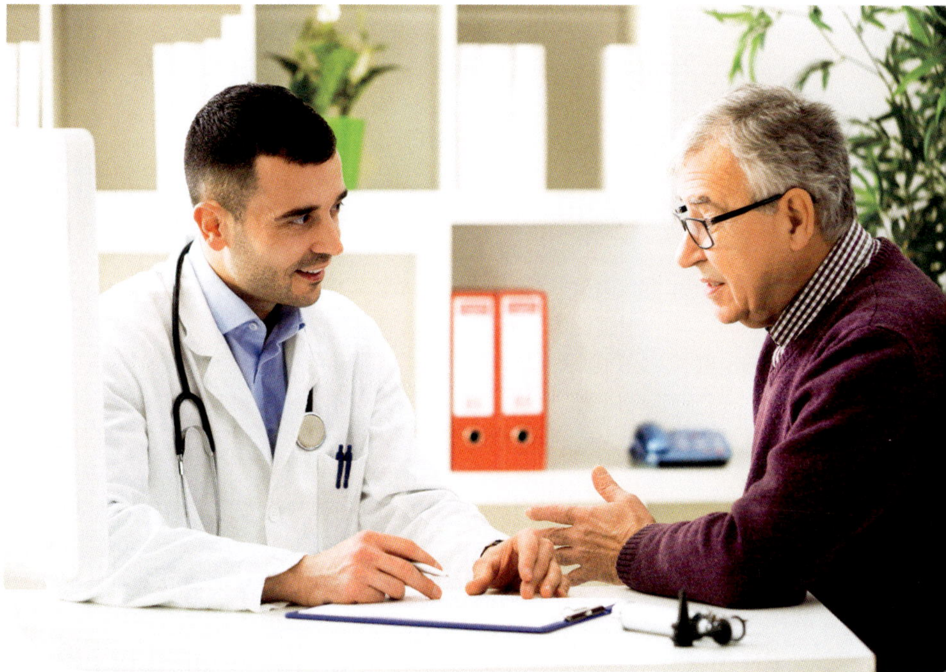

lives as they come in for appointments. He builds trust with them through years of care.

## WHAT IS A PHYSICIAN ASSISTANT?

A PA works with physicians, who are also called doctors. A PA may help a doctor with medical procedures. PAs also work on their own. They examine patients and prescribe medication. The doctor may be their supervisor or work partner.

Both PAs and doctors must have a master's degree. But doctors have more training and education. They can do more medical tasks and procedures. For example, doctors can lead surgeries. A PA can assist a surgeon with surgery. But they are not allowed to lead surgery. And a PA must have a doctor in the operating room with them.

A PA can do other medical tasks. They can order tests. They can stitch cuts or freeze off warts. They may also do lab research. It does not take as long to become a PA as it does to become a doctor. That means a PA can start their career sooner than a doctor can.

PAs may check a patient's blood pressure.

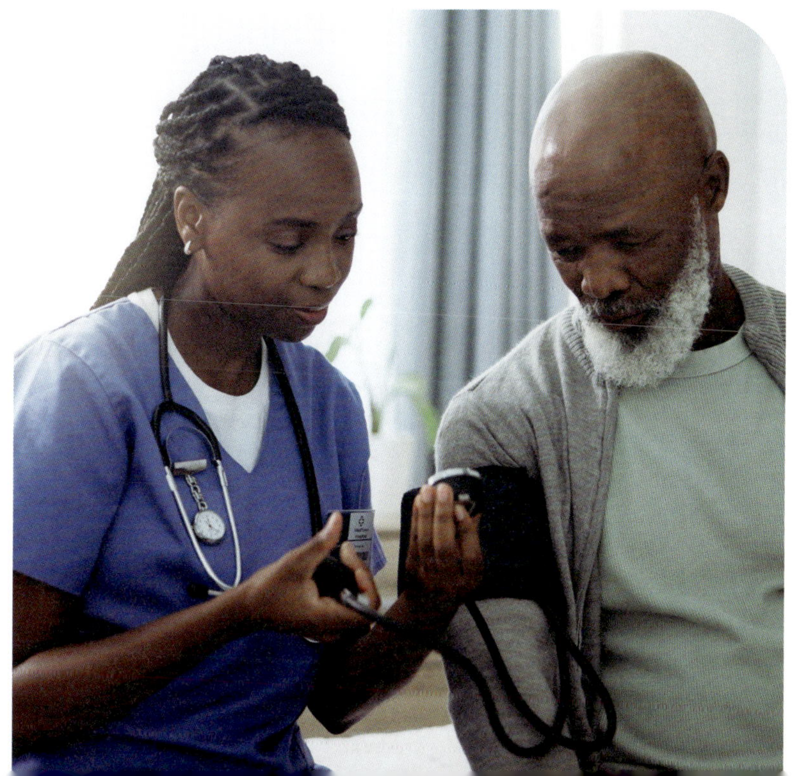

# WHAT DOES A PHYSICIAN ASSISTANT DO?

One of a PA's tasks is to keep records of a patient's medical history. Medical histories are documents. They include information about a patient's health. This includes past diseases and other health issues. Doctors review these notes. Medical histories help give a patient more personalized treatment. For example, a patient's medical history includes allergies. This can prevent a PA from prescribing

PAs make sure a patient's medical needs are met.

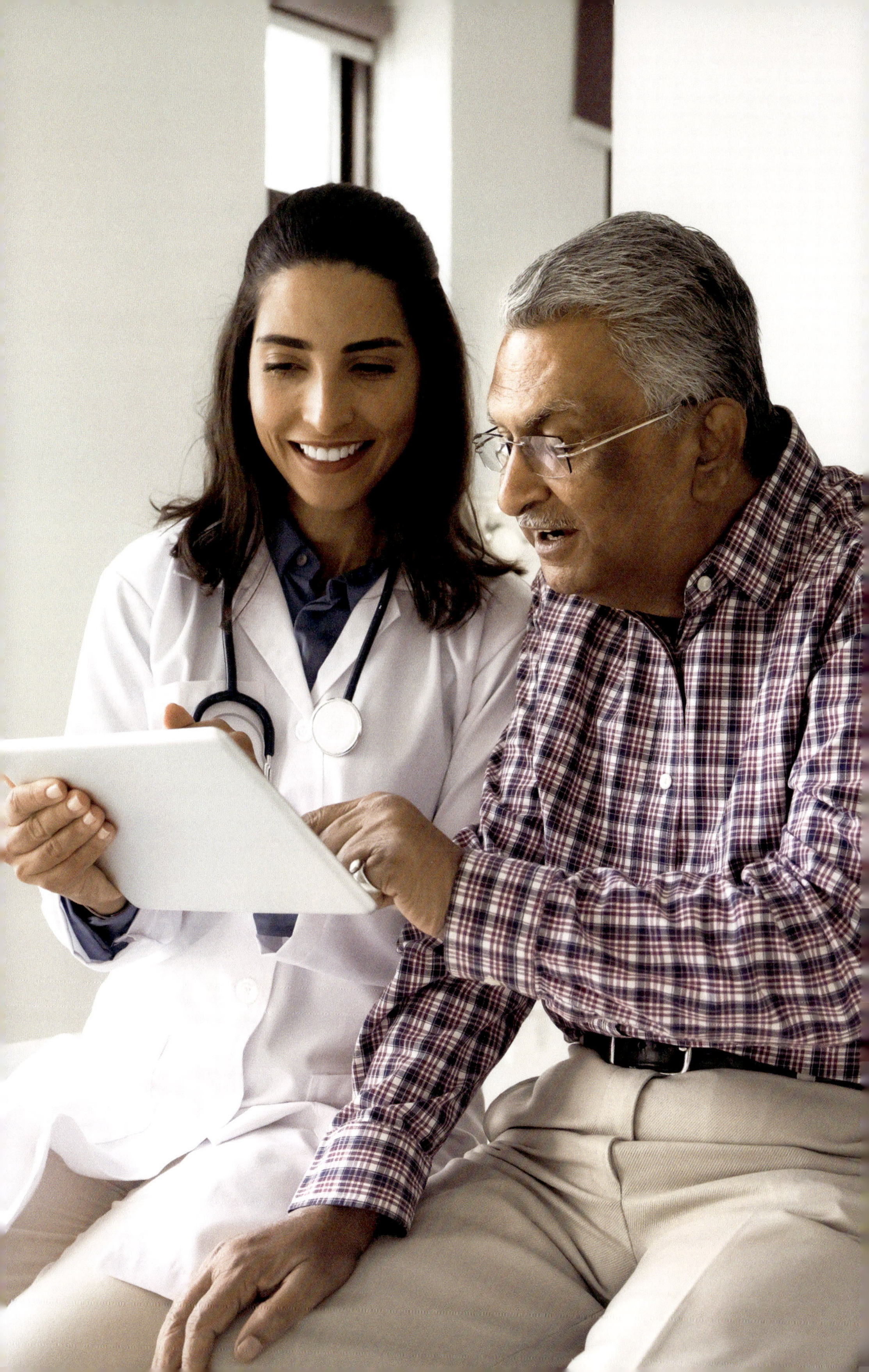

medicine to that patient that could cause an allergic reaction.

PAs examine patients to see if they are healthy. They diagnose medical conditions. This means they look for what may be causing problems for the patient. Knowing the cause is the first step in treating health issues. PAs order medical tests. These include blood tests or X-rays. They study the patient's test results. Then they can prescribe medication for the patient.

PAs continue to learn about medical discoveries in their field. Some PAs may do research in a lab. They study different types of diseases.

Some PAs work in operating rooms. They help with surgeries. PAs make sure the surgeon has the correct tools

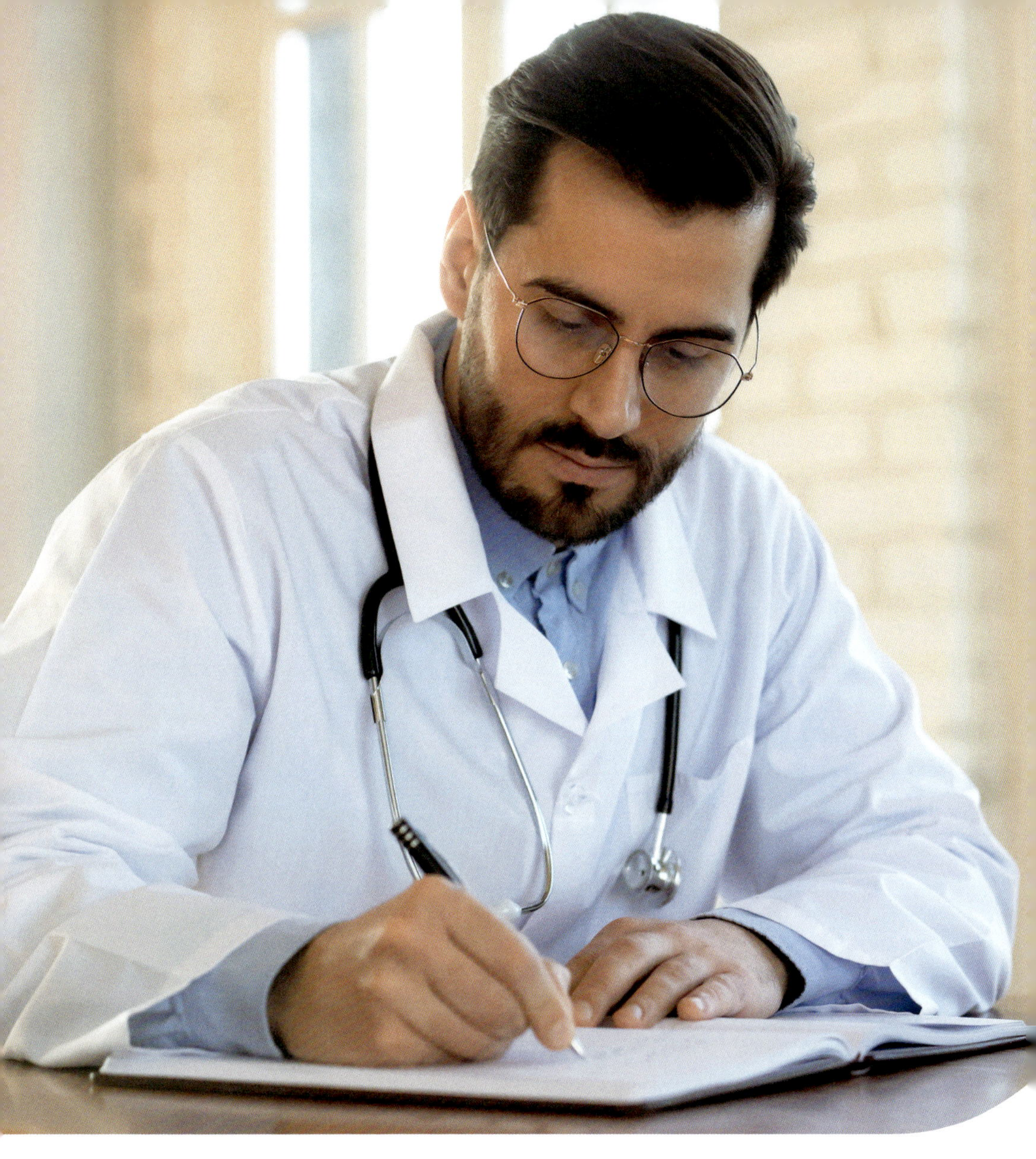

**PAs must keep up to date on medical studies that could affect their patients.**

and supplies needed. Surgical PAs can insert tubes to help patients breathe during surgery.

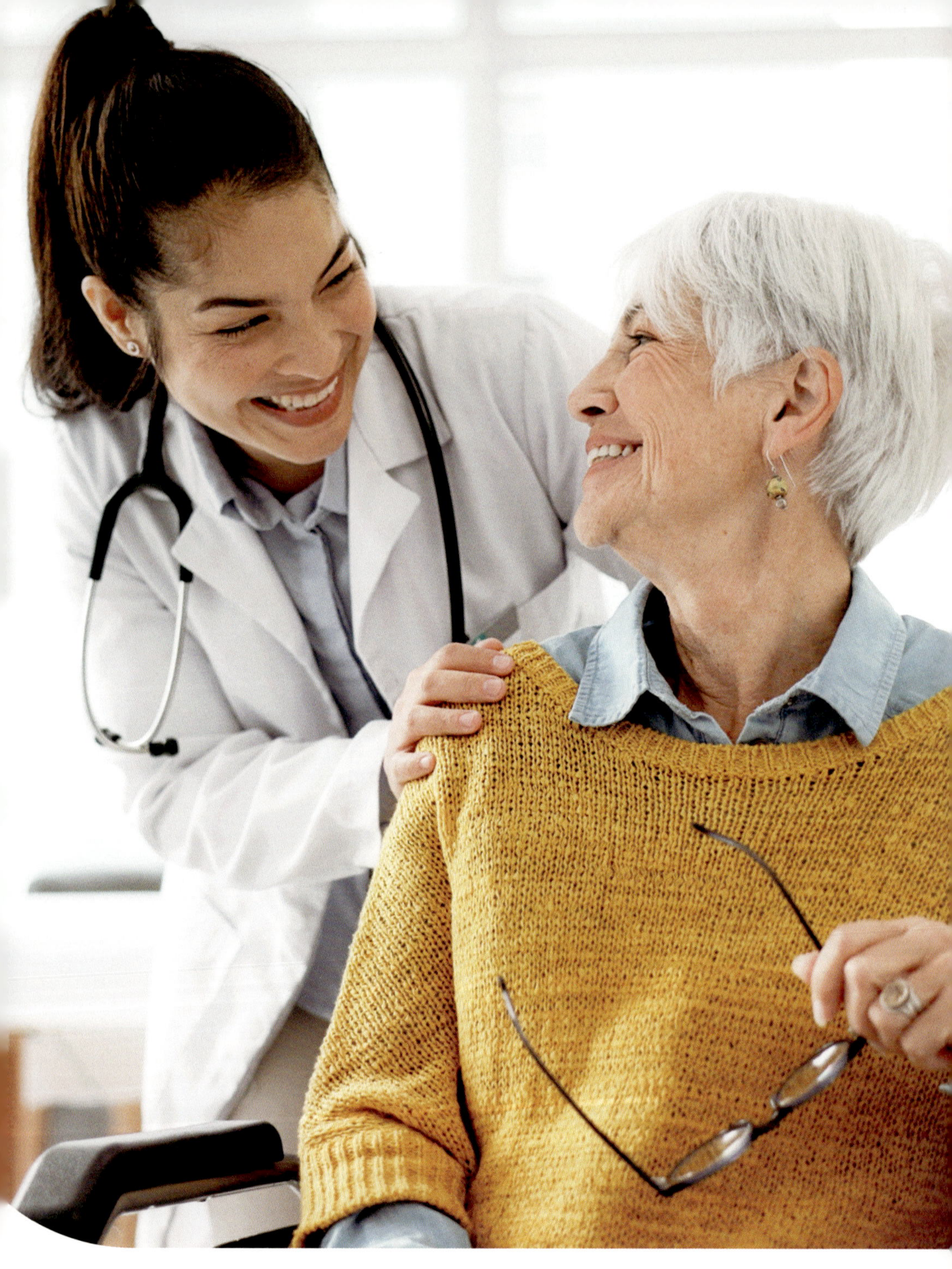

PAs work hard to make sure all patients get the best quality care.

PAs teach patients how to take care of their health. That might include ways to eat a healthy diet. PAs might give a patient information on how to stop smoking. If a patient sprains their ankle, the PA can provide a care plan for healing. It might include rest, keeping the foot **elevated**, and icing the ankle. PA Amber Davis says,

> *It's extremely rewarding to see a patient make progress. Whether they quit smoking, lower weight, lower their blood sugar, or make some other positive change, I get to see it and celebrate it with them at follow-up appointments.*[1]

PAs can become leaders in their field. They may manage medical employees at hospitals and clinics. This includes nurses and new PAs. They may teach other PAs in the field. PAs might also run their own health care business. They can even lead a team of medical researchers.

## DIFFERENT PA SPECIALTIES

There are many types of PAs. Some PAs choose to specialize. These PAs focus on a specific area of medicine. They gain additional skills for the role. As the Mayo Clinic explains,

> *Because PAs have the opportunity to excel in virtually any specialty area of medicine, types of physician assistants span a variety of roles, specialties, and sub-specialty areas. PAs have the ability to specialize in one or several areas throughout their career.*[2]

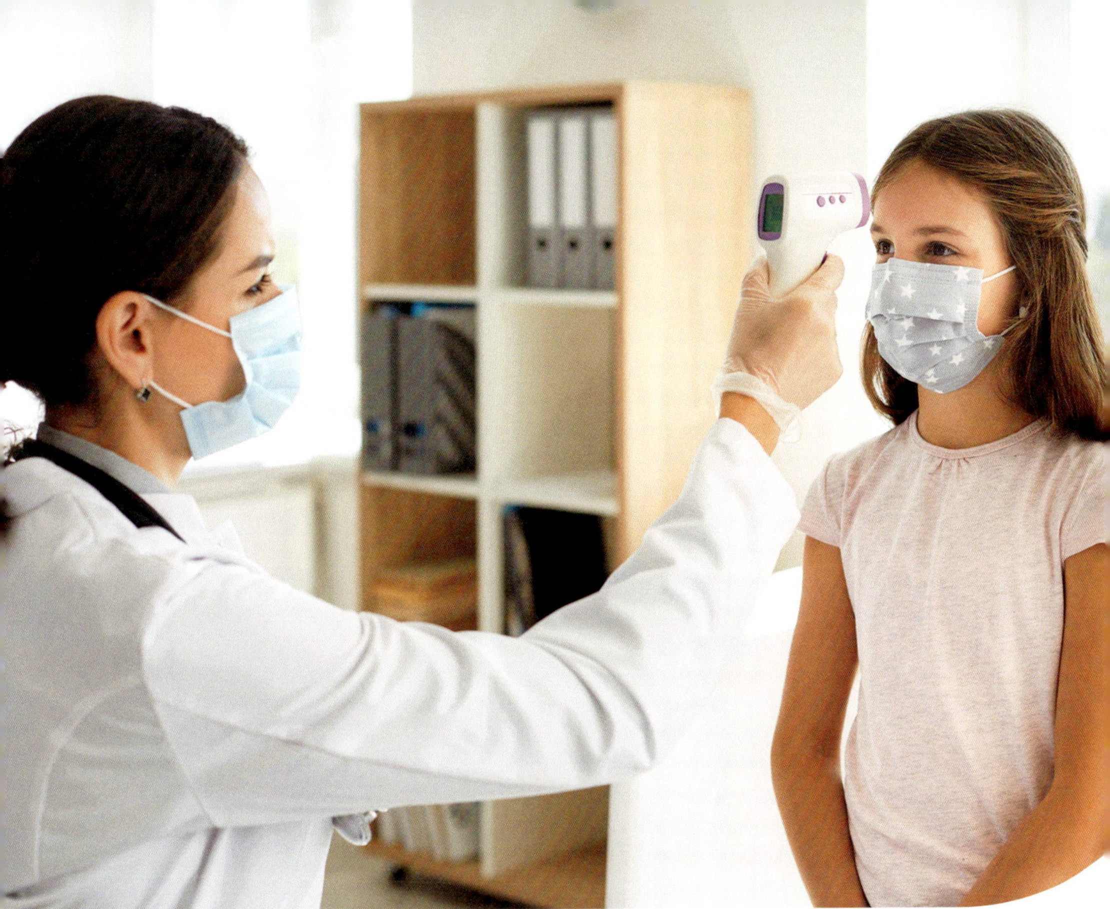

**Thermometers are used to check a patient's body temperature.**

For example, a PA might specialize in cardiac care. They help keep the heart strong. They examine a person's heart rate and blood pressure. They check a patient's family history of heart attacks.

Other PAs may work in primary care. They work with a wide range of health

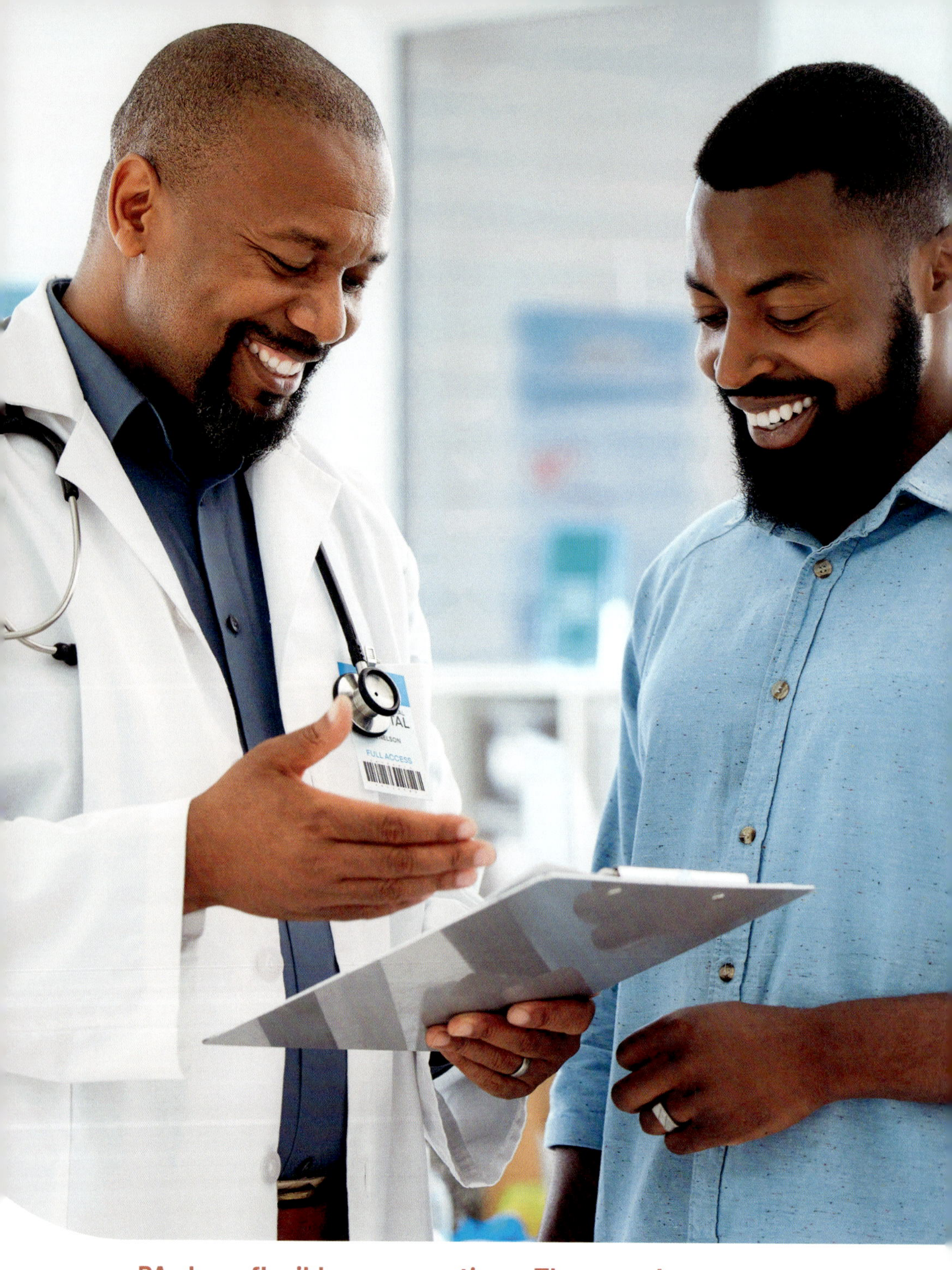


PAs have flexible career options. They can do many different tasks.

conditions. They help prevent, diagnose, and treat illnesses. They may test someone for strep throat. They help with injuries, too. This includes small scrapes and cuts. Sometimes a patient needs more advanced care. A primary care PA can help them find a specialist to care for them.

Some PAs specialize in emergency medicine. This field focuses on severe or sudden accidents and illnesses. People who are badly hurt often go to emergency rooms (ERs). PAs who work in ERs are trained to handle different emergencies. Treatment must be done quickly. PAs apply pressure to stop bleeding. They set broken bones. They prepare patients for surgery if needed.

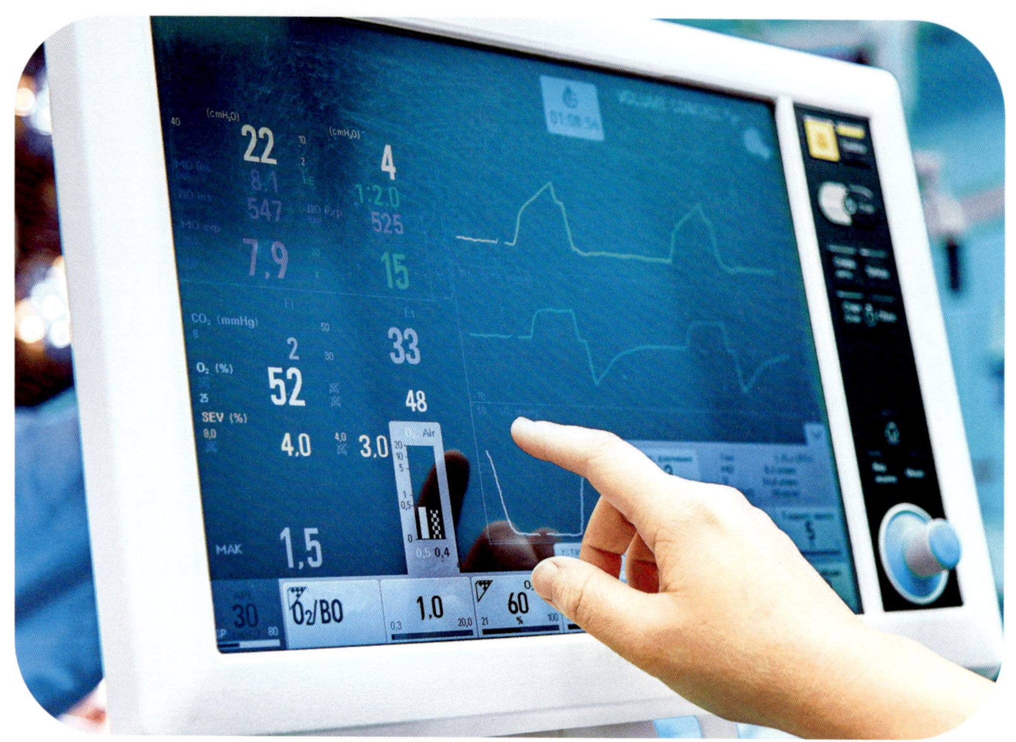


**PAs may help monitor vital signs during surgery.**

Some PAs specialize in pediatrics. This field focuses on infants, children, and young adults. They work with pediatricians. These are physicians who specialize in this area, too.

Pediatric PAs have to complete additional training. They may help doctors with routine checkups. They may ask parents questions about a child's physical activity and healthy eating habits. They measure the child's weight and height. They give vaccines and other needed shots.

Some PAs specialize in **rheumatology**. They help reduce patient pain. They help patients experiencing numbness, too. This may affect places such as the shoulders, wrists, and knees. PAs review health records and conduct tests on potential problem areas. They order X-rays. They also provide patients with ways to reduce pain such as medicine and exercises.

## WHERE A PA WORKS

PAs work in doctor's offices, clinics, and hospitals. They also work in nursing homes. PAs may treat patients in small examination rooms. These rooms usually include an exam table for tools. They also have a sink with soap for the PA to **sanitize** their hands.

PAs can also visit nursing homes. They meet different patients. Some PAs work in geriatrics. This medical field focuses on working with older people. These PAs may work at nursing homes where medical professionals are on staff. PAs do follow-up visits to check on patients who have been ill

## Radiology

Radiology is an area of medicine. It involves using tools such as X-rays and other imaging devices. It lets medical professionals see inside a patient's body. X-rays can detect broken bones, heart problems, and diseases. This includes cancer.

or injured. Some PAs work full-time at one nursing home. PAs can meet with families of residents to discuss the resident's needs.

Sadie Siarkiewicz is a PA who works with people who are aging. She says,

> *I . . . started working on a memory care unit. I had no idea that that position would change my life forever. My residents and their families became my second family. . . . This is where my passion for the geriatric population started, and I knew I wanted to make a difference.*[3]

PAs can join the military. This includes the US Army, Navy, Air Force, Coast Guard, and National Guard. They work at military bases and provide service to military members. They also work at US

## PA AVERAGE INCOME

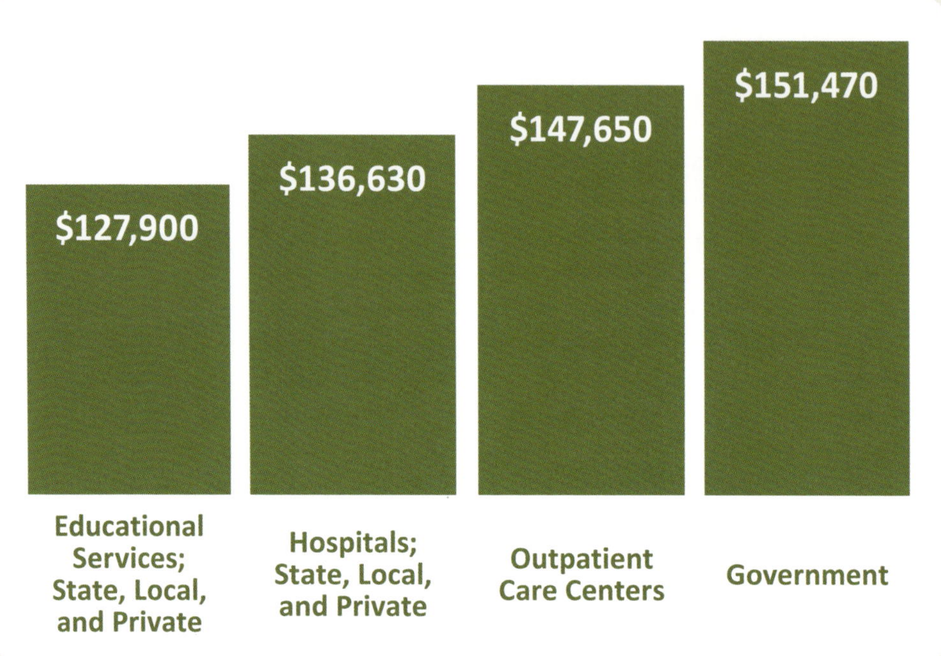


*Source: "Occupational Outlook Handbook: Physician Assistants,"* US Bureau of Labor Statistics, *April 18, 2025. www.bls.gov.*

**A PA's income may depend on where they work. This graph shows the average income earned in different industries.**

Department of Veterans Affairs (VA) clinics and hospitals. The VA is a government organization. It works with military members and veterans. The VA has many clinics and hospitals. Primary care and specialist PAs work for the VA.

**VA clinics and hospitals provide veterans with health care services such as mental health programs.**

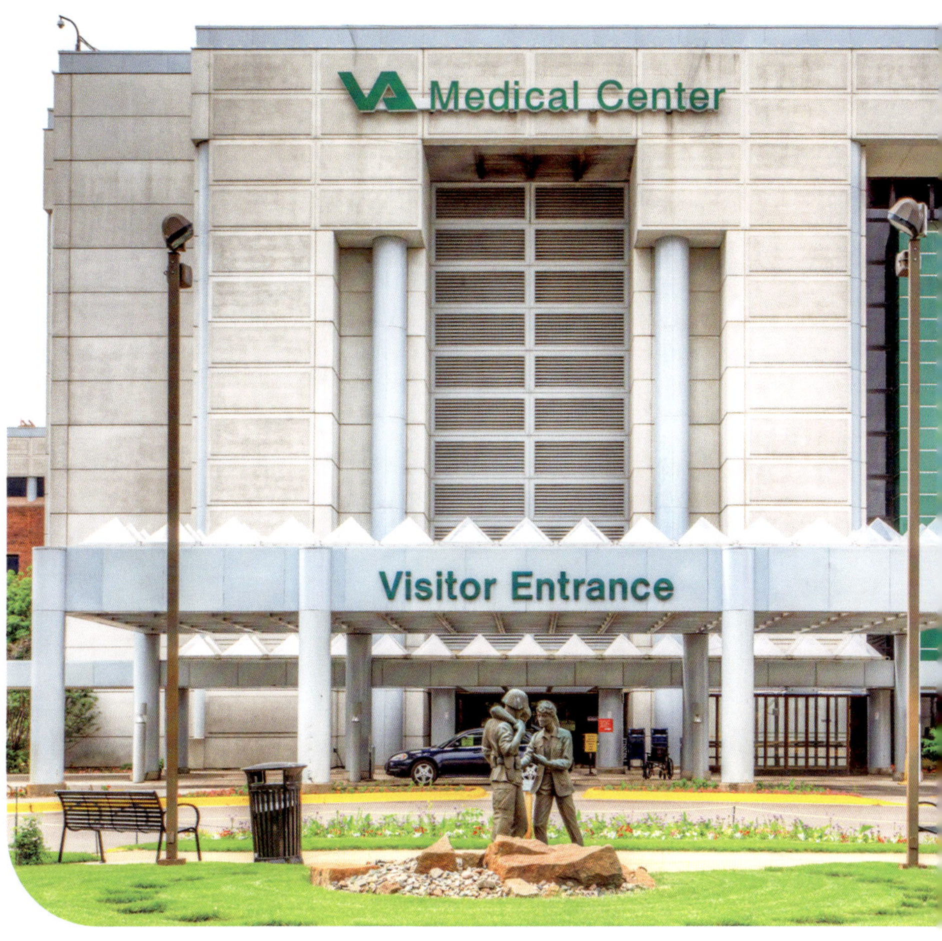

# CHAPTER TWO

# BECOMING A PHYSICIAN ASSISTANT

The first step to becoming a PA is to earn an undergraduate degree. Students attend a college or university for about 4 years. Students should focus on the sciences. This can include biology, which is the study of living things. Other students study psychology. This is the study of the human mind and how it works.

Some schools offer a pre-PA track. Students who want to become a PA may

**Students interested in becoming PAs may take classes that have lectures and labs. Labs provide students with practical skills.**

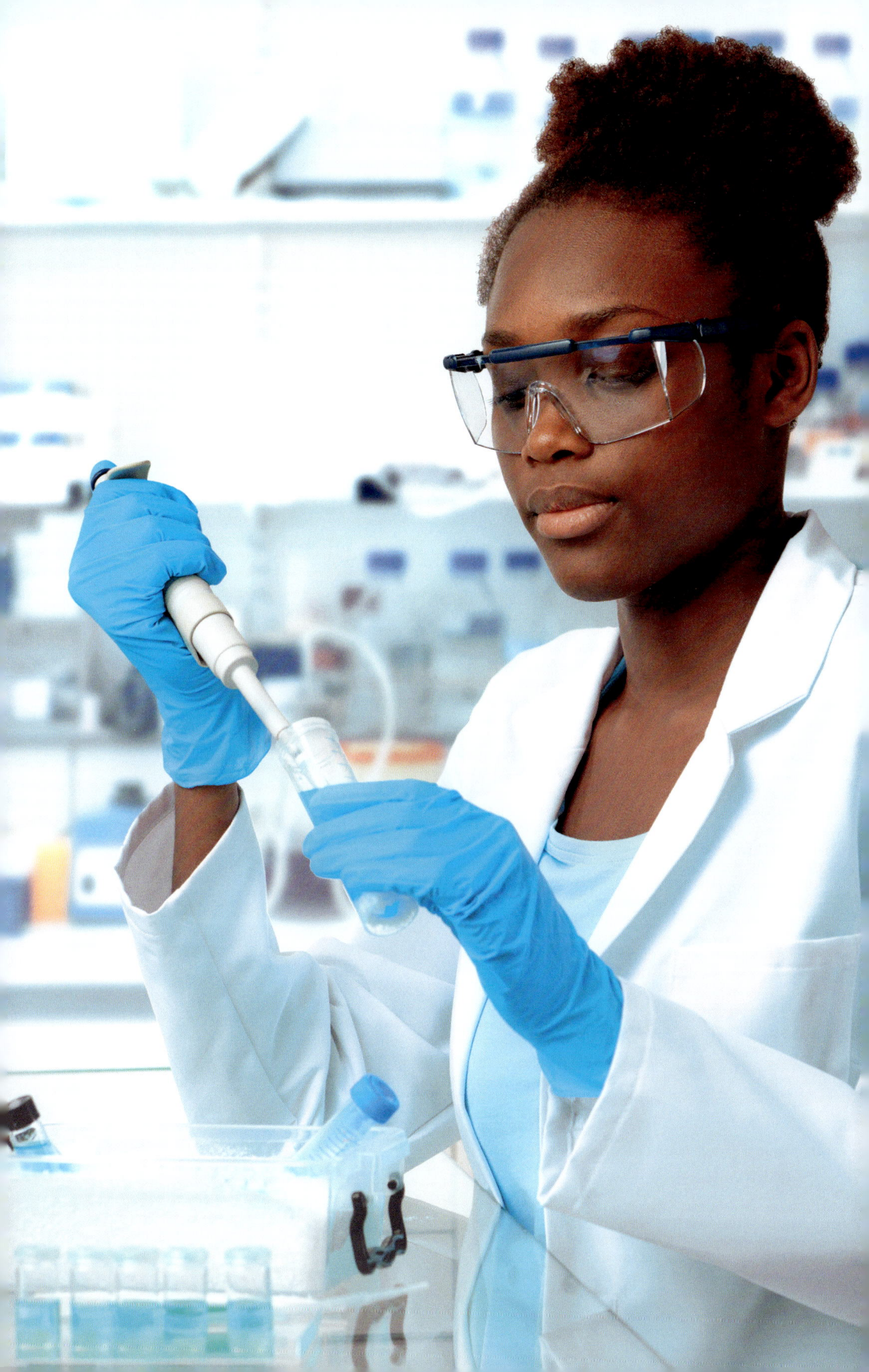

choose this program. It is not a degree. But it prepares students for PA school. The program teaches students about human health and wellness.

After students complete their undergraduate degree, they must enter an accredited PA course. Accreditation shows

**Study groups can help students learn, allowing them to talk through difficult questions.**

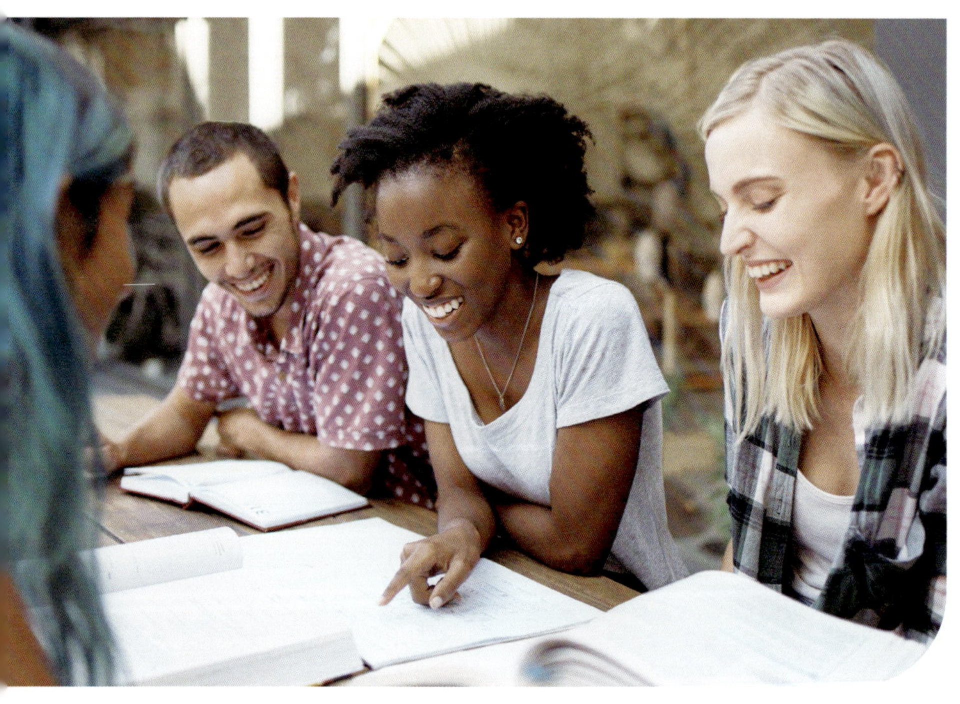

that a school offers a good-quality program. It is done by an organization called the Accreditation Review Commission on Education for the Physician Assistant. PA programs last at least 2 years.

## STEPS TO A PA CAREER

PA programs are **rigorous**. For PAs, classroom learning includes many kinds of science courses. Some are required for all medical professionals. This includes anatomy. It is the study of the structure and parts of the human body. Students study things such as muscle and tissue groups.

PA students also study genetics. This is the study of how certain traits are passed from parent to child. Students will study different medical **terminology** as well.

PA student programs include classroom learning and clinical rotations.

Clinical rotations help students learn how to apply classroom learning to real-life patients. PA students may practice diagnosing patients. They may educate patients about health conditions. They learn to communicate with patients. PAs must be able to write and update medical histories. As student PAs, they will take many writing courses to help with communication tasks.

During clinical rotations, a preceptor helps supervise PA students. Preceptors are people with experience in the medical field. They find medical opportunities for students to practice. A preceptor also provides PA students with helpful feedback. PAs then apply these notes for the next

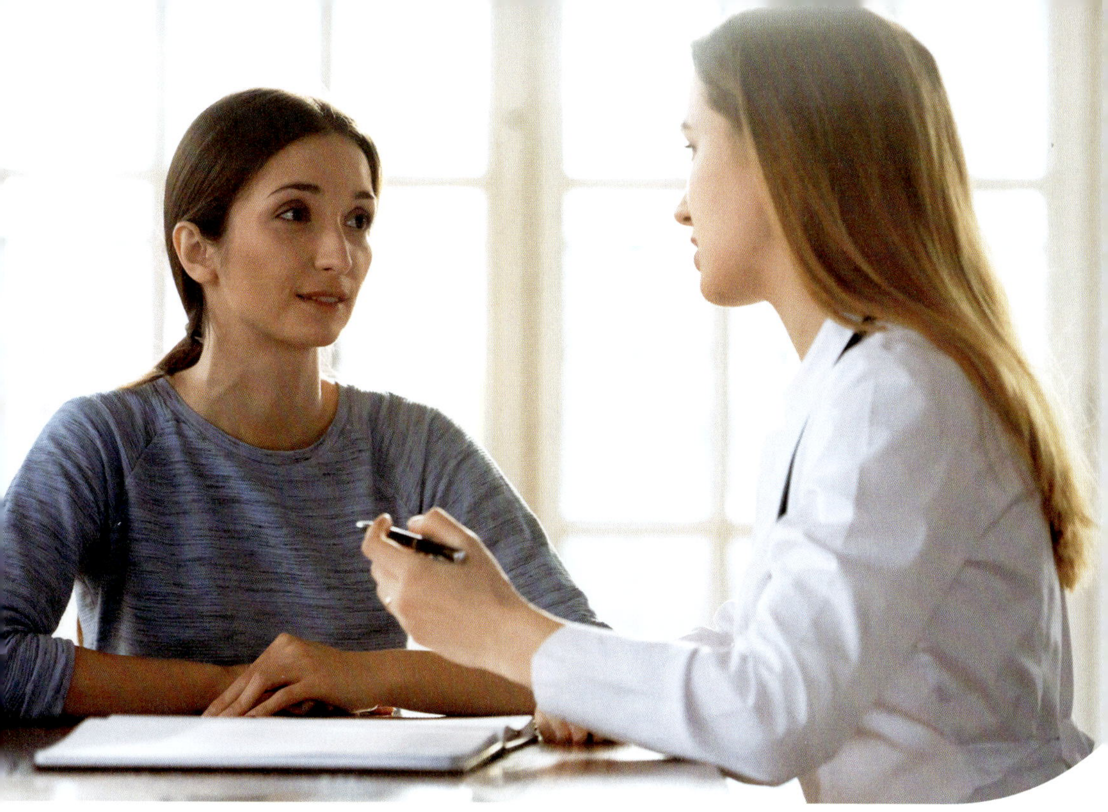

**PAs must have excellent communication skills. They must learn how to respond to patients and actively listen.**

clinical rotation. If PAs have any questions, preceptors are useful resources.

Clinical rotations help PA students gain experience. They may work in a hospital, clinic, or nursing home. They may try primary care or other specialties. This helps PAs decide if they want to become specialists. PA Diana Anderson said,

*When rotations started, I knew I was interested in emergency medicine but I tried my best to keep an open mind. I ended up loving every single rotation and truly could see myself practicing in all areas of medicine. Ultimately, I landed my very first job in urgent care.*[4]

**PAs who work at nursing homes help monitor patient health. They also write care plans.**

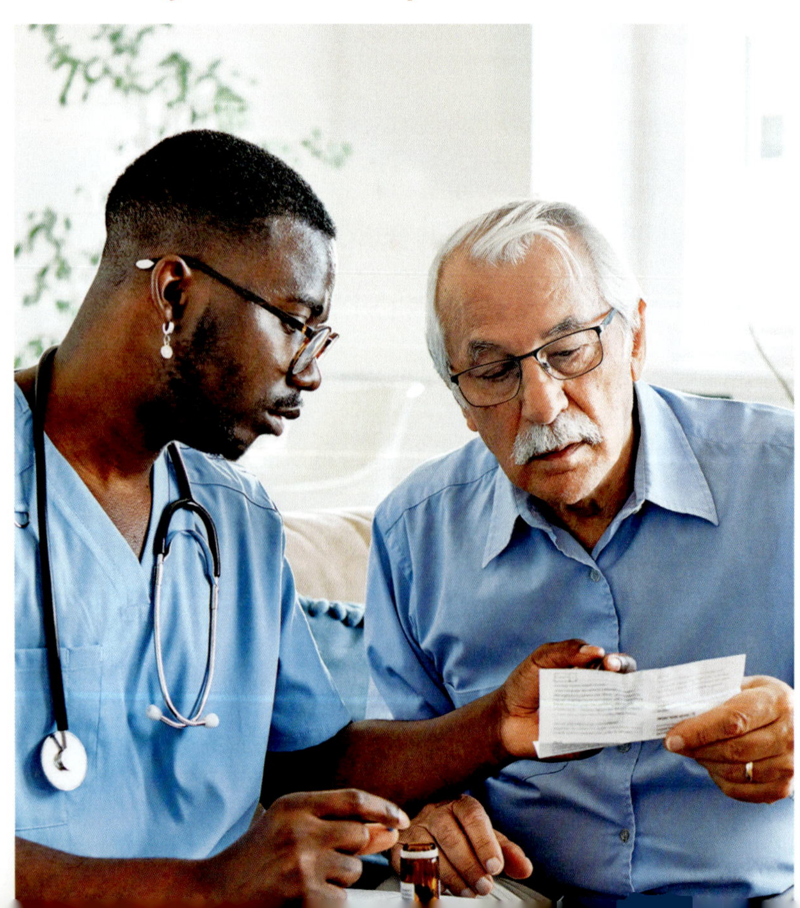

## LICENSURE AND CERTIFICATION

The next step for PAs is to become certified. A professional group verifies that PAs meet the requirements. In the United States, the group is called the National Commission on Certification of Physician Assistants (NCCPA).

The NCCPA offers the Physician Assistant National Certifying Exam (PANCE).

### Other Medical Degrees

A PA may choose to earn another degree. Their decision may depend on if they want to change careers or do research. A doctor of medicine (MD) degree is required to become a doctor. An MD-PhD is for someone who wants to be a doctor and a researcher or scientist. A degree may increase the amount of money someone makes.

PAs must pass the test to become certified. The test asks questions about procedures and different causes of illness. It also asks about what different symptoms might mean. There are 300 multiple-choice questions.

Once PAs are certified, they must keep their certification current. This means they must complete at least 100 hours of continuing medical education. They do this every 2 years. They also recertify every 10 years.

Finally, PAs must apply for a license. This is proof that PAs have completed the required training and education. It also shows that they passed a licensure exam.

PAs must have a license from the state in which they will work. To get the license approved, PAs must have passed the

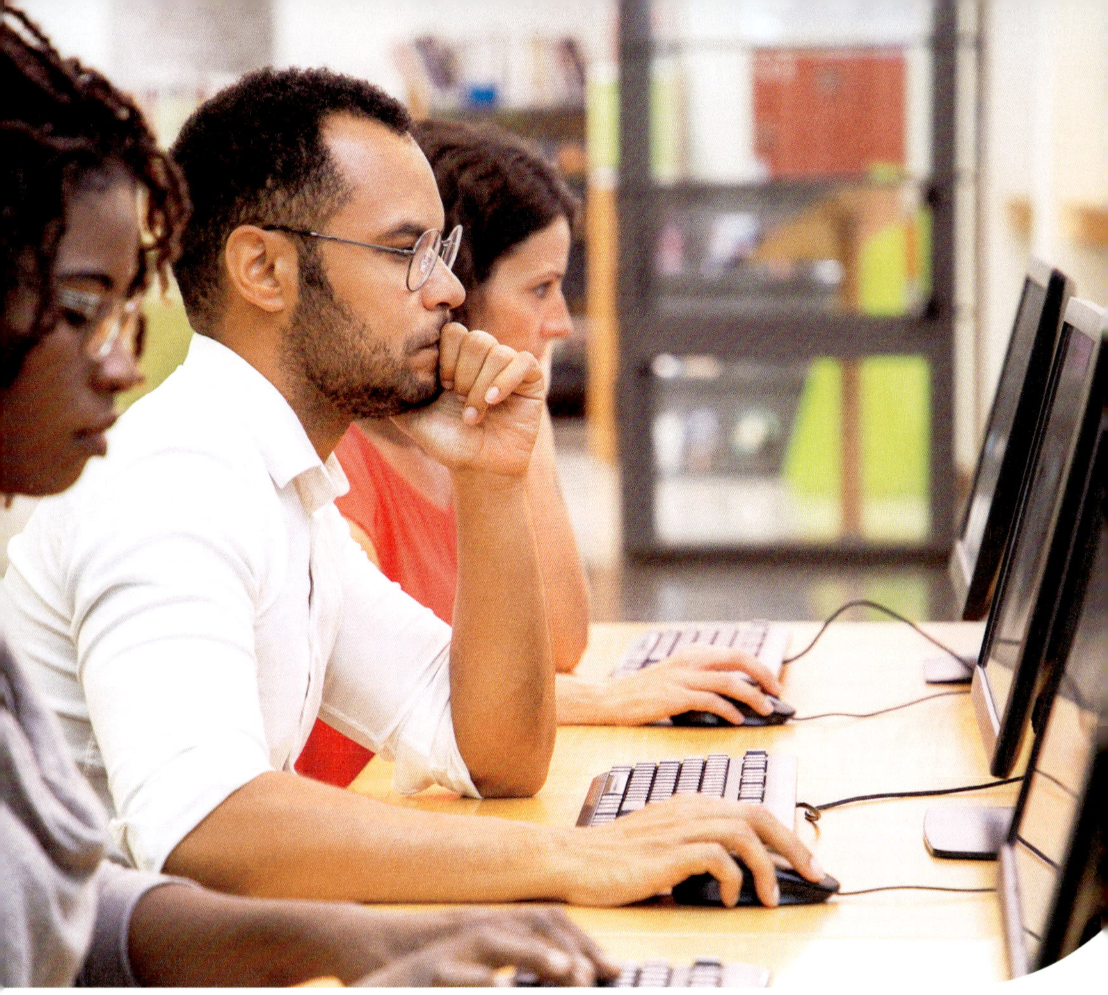

**The Physician Assistant National Certifying Exam is a timed test. The exam lasts 5 hours in total.**

certification exam. Licenses are granted by government **agencies**. It is hard work to become a PA. But the career provides many opportunities for those who want to support patients in the health care profession.

# CHAPTER THREE

# A DAY IN THE LIFE OF A PHYSICIAN ASSISTANT

Physician assistants work in many places. They have different responsibilities depending on their specialty and where they work. Some work with patients of all ages. Others may work only with children or older people.

This means there is not one typical workday for PAs. But all PAs share common tasks. They meet with patients. They diagnose problems and suggest treatments.

**PAs may work on call. This means they are called into work outside of their scheduled hours.**

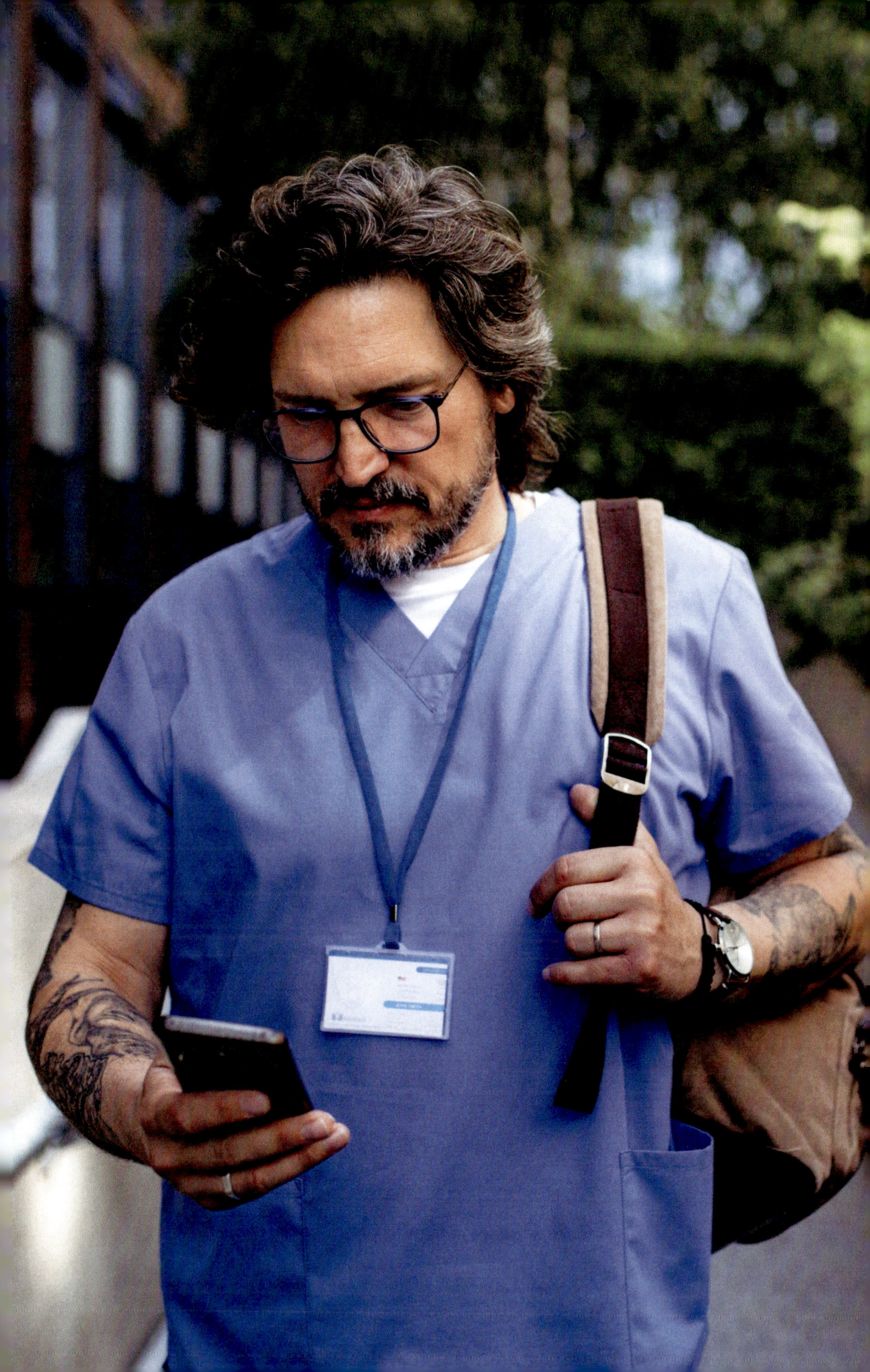

## PRIMARY CARE PA

At a primary care clinic, the day begins early. The PA may have to be at the office by 7:00 a.m. They use a computer to check for new messages. This could include lab test results and patient questions.

Then the PA begins seeing patients. They meet with as many as twenty-five patients in one day. Each appointment lasts between

### When PAs Work

PAs have many different work schedules. Those who work in primary care offices usually work weekdays from 7:00 a.m. to 5:00 p.m. But PAs who work in hospitals or other locations have different hours. They may work nights or weekends. They may also have to work federal holidays, including the Fourth of July or Thanksgiving.

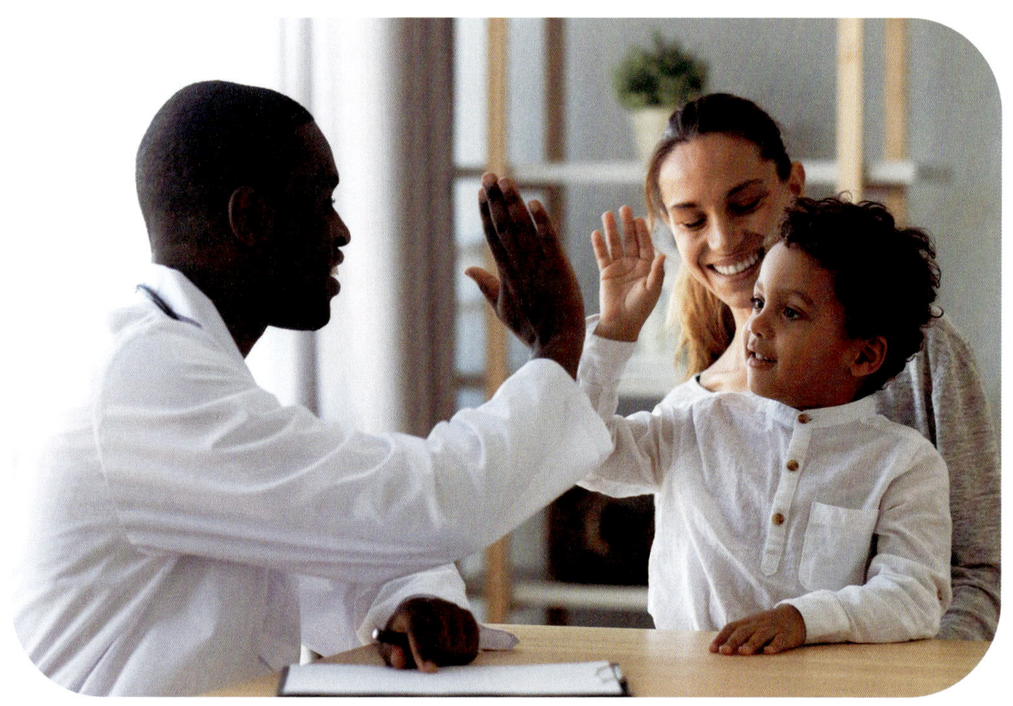

**PAs who work at hospitals may meet with 50 patients or more in a week.**

15 and 30 minutes. This includes quick follow-up visits. PAs check in with patients they have seen recently about a health issue. They make sure the patient is doing better. Some patients may need longer appointments. For example, a physical is an exam that checks on a person's general health. Other patients need medical procedures. This includes getting stitches.

PAs have many other kinds of appointments, too. They may examine a child who wants to play a sport and needs proof of good health. They provide shots that help patients with pain. They may remove an unusual mole on the skin. Then they may send it out for a biopsy. A biopsy is a lab test of body tissue. PAs sometimes see patients who are mostly healthy. They may need advice about diet and exercise. As the day goes on, PAs might take time to answer emails. They also take a short lunch break.

One benefit of working in primary care is getting to know the patients. People return to see the same PA. The PA gets to know them well. One PA said, "My favorite aspect of family medicine is getting to

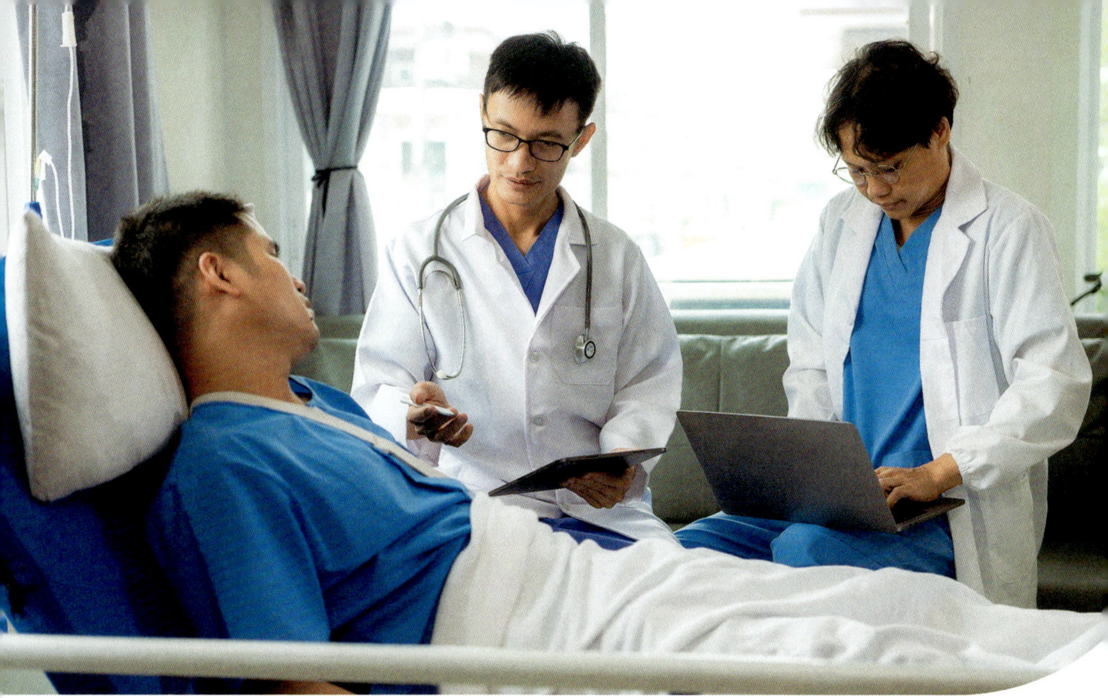

**PAs ask a series of questions to patients. This helps them accurately diagnose illnesses.**

know my patients. . . . This is something I cherished, and you don't get it in many specialties."[5]

## INTERNAL MEDICINE PA

Internal medicine PAs examine, diagnose, and treat conditions in adults. In the hospital, they will treat patients who are injured or ill. Sometimes they work in the ER. This means they have to adapt to

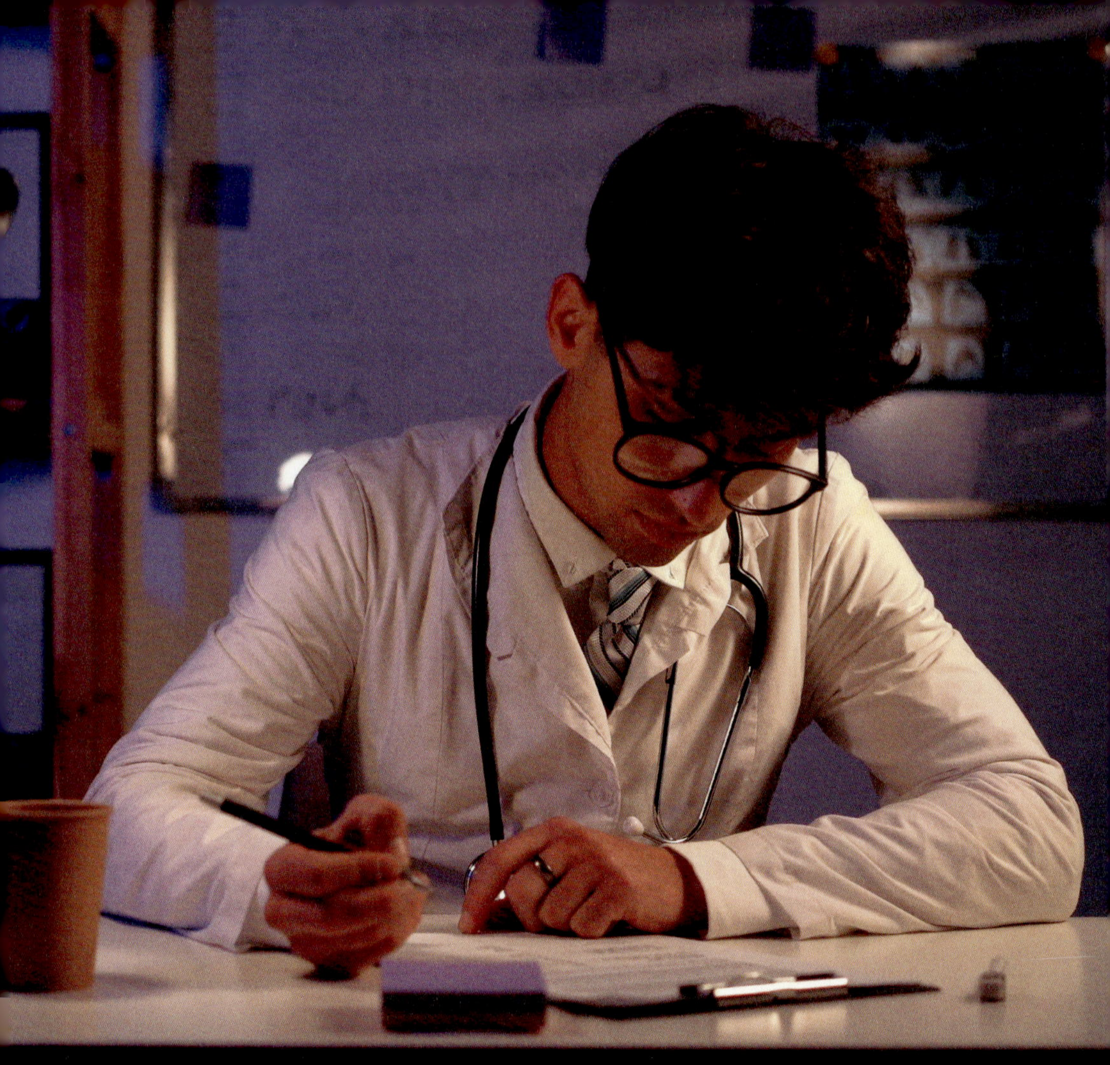

**PAs may work night shifts. They monitor and care for patients who have health issues during the night.**

fast-paced work environments. They learn to multitask. It can be stressful, but PAs work together to support each other.

PAs who work at hospitals may start their day as early as 6:00 a.m. Other PAs start in the afternoon and work late into the evening. A typical shift can last 12 hours.

In the morning, PAs go on rounds with a doctor. Rounds take place once a day. The doctor will take a team to visit different patients. The team could include PAs, nurses, and pharmacists. A pharmacist is a health care professional who works with medicine. The team might also include a physical therapist (PT). A PT is a specialist who helps patients recover from injuries such as a pulled muscle.

Members of this team talk to the patients about their health conditions. They will also discuss next steps. That may include more tests, surgery, or other treatments.

Adrijana Anderson is a PA who works in internal medicine. She loves going on rounds. She says,

> *These rounds are one of the best parts about working in the* ***ICU****. It is a great way to improve communication and prevent errors in patient care. . . . We are all better providers because of this* ***collaboration****.*[6]

At night, PAs may work with patients who have been admitted to the hospital. These patients may need extra support and care. PAs may need to give patients medicine in the middle of the night. PAs and other medical staff work together to meet patient needs. It is hard work, but PAs get an opportunity to take care of patients from many backgrounds.

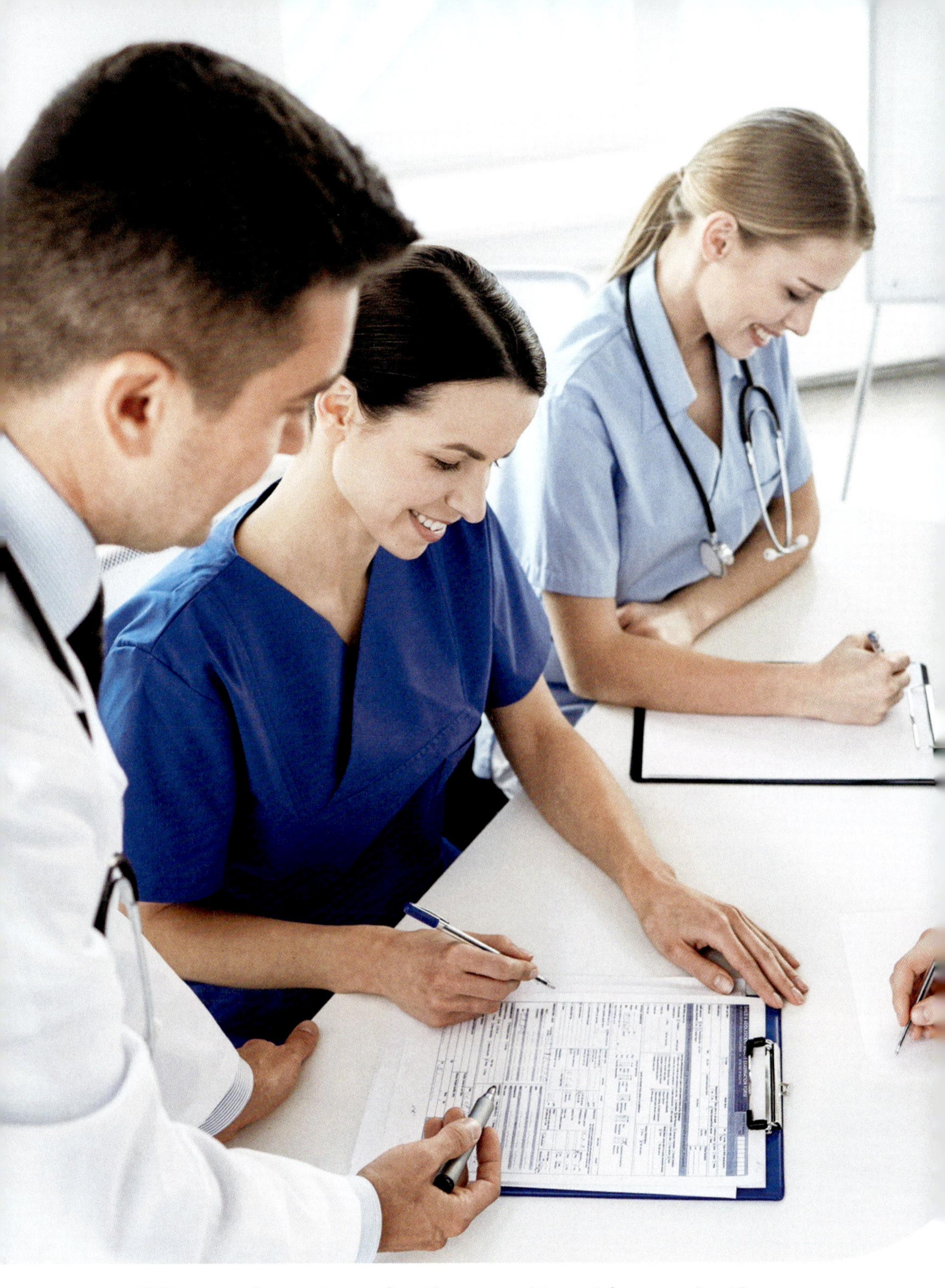

PAs are always learning from and teaching each other.

# THE OUTLOOK FOR PHYSICIAN ASSISTANTS

The US Bureau of Labor Statistics (BLS) is a government agency. It gathers different information about careers. This includes information about the income people earn in different types of careers and workplaces.

The BLS predicted that PA jobs will increase 28 percent between 2023 and 2033. Other jobs are expected to grow only 4 percent during that time. This means

**PAs play an important role in keeping communities healthy.**

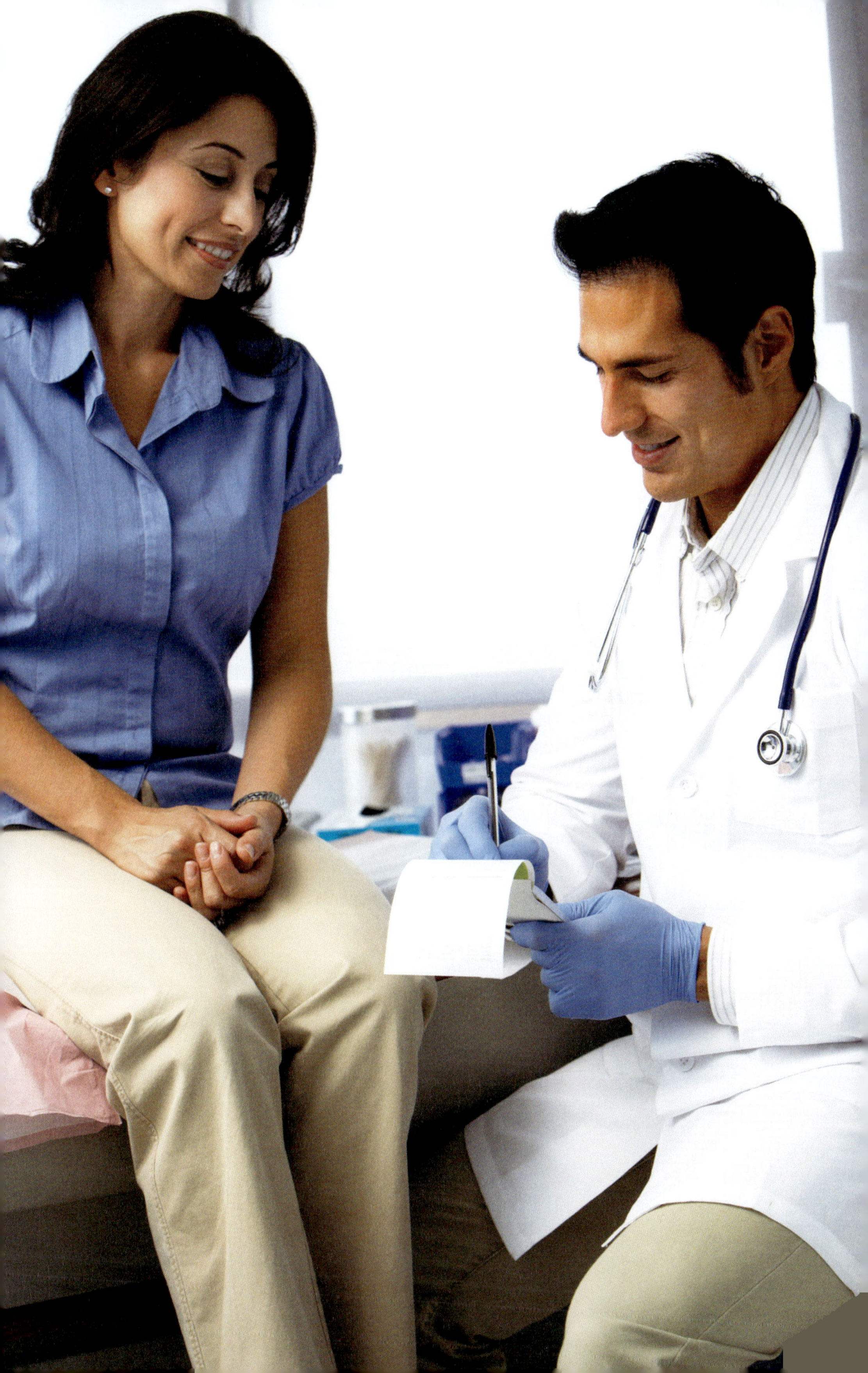

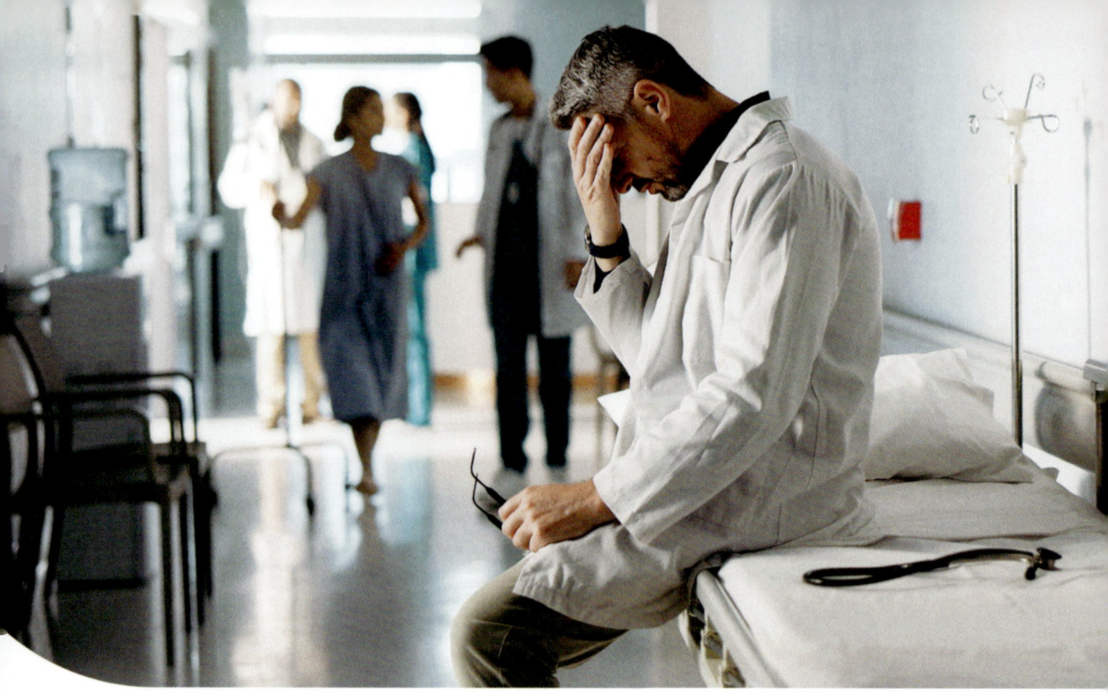

**PAs practice self-care to prevent burnout. This may include taking deep breaths or taking a break.**

there will be many PA jobs available in the future.

## REASONS FOR HIGH GROWTH

There are many reasons why the BLS expects the PA field to grow. One is that many people in the United States are growing older. As people age, they often need more medical care. The number of people with ongoing illnesses may also increase. This includes people with diseases such as diabetes. They will need additional medical care.

PAs can perform many of the same duties as doctors. But they do not have to go to school as long. That means they can begin working sooner.

PAs are also in demand for team-based health care. This means they may work together with other health care staff to take care of different patients. By spreading out patient care, PAs make sure that patients get the attention they need. PAs are better able to provide individual support, too. PAs may also face less stress as they have a larger team to assist them.

PAs have flexible careers. They can work in different facilities. PAs can also have different specializations. That means that PAs have many job opportunities. If they do not like their current job, there are likely others they can move into.

## FUTURE GROWTH

Some states are allowing experienced PAs to handle more responsibilities. They may work on their own without supervision from a doctor. This could help provide more care in smaller communities, increasing access to health care.

Technology is another factor in future demand. Improvements to technology make it easier for PAs to practice medicine online. PAs are trained to use telehealth to help patients. This allows PAs and patients to meet remotely using computers.

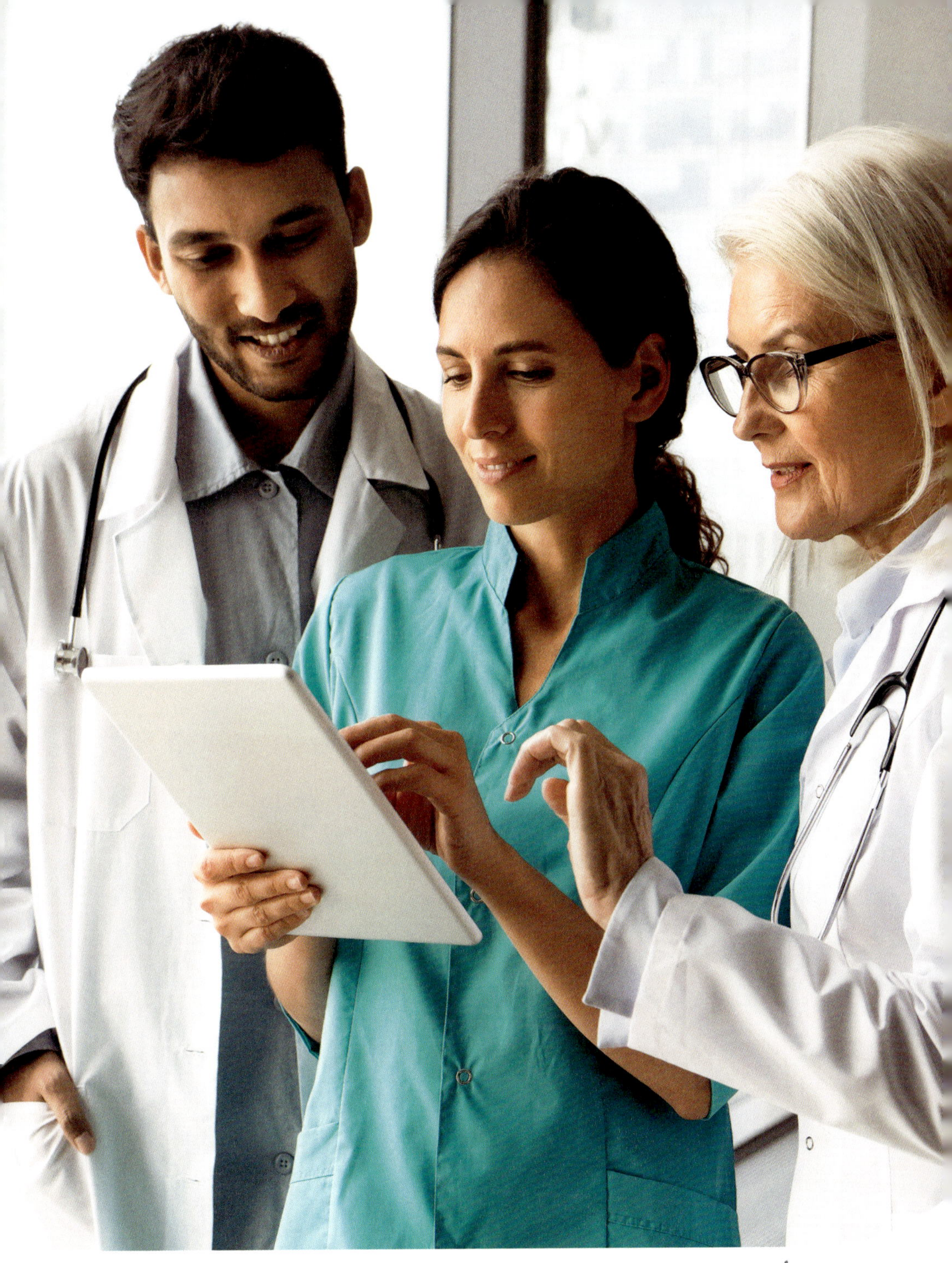

A team of different health care professionals helps provide better care for patients.

PAs help answer questions. They also help with ongoing issues such as high blood pressure.

Artificial intelligence (AI) may help PAs diagnose conditions quickly and accurately. That means patients may be diagnosed sooner. They can also begin treatment earlier. AI may help PAs develop patient care plans. This would allow PAs to spend more time with patients.

Today, PAs have more opportunities to work in various fields. They can start in a general practice providing primary care. They do many types of tasks. But they have other options, too.

PAs could receive training to take on leadership roles. They could go back to graduate school to learn a specialty.

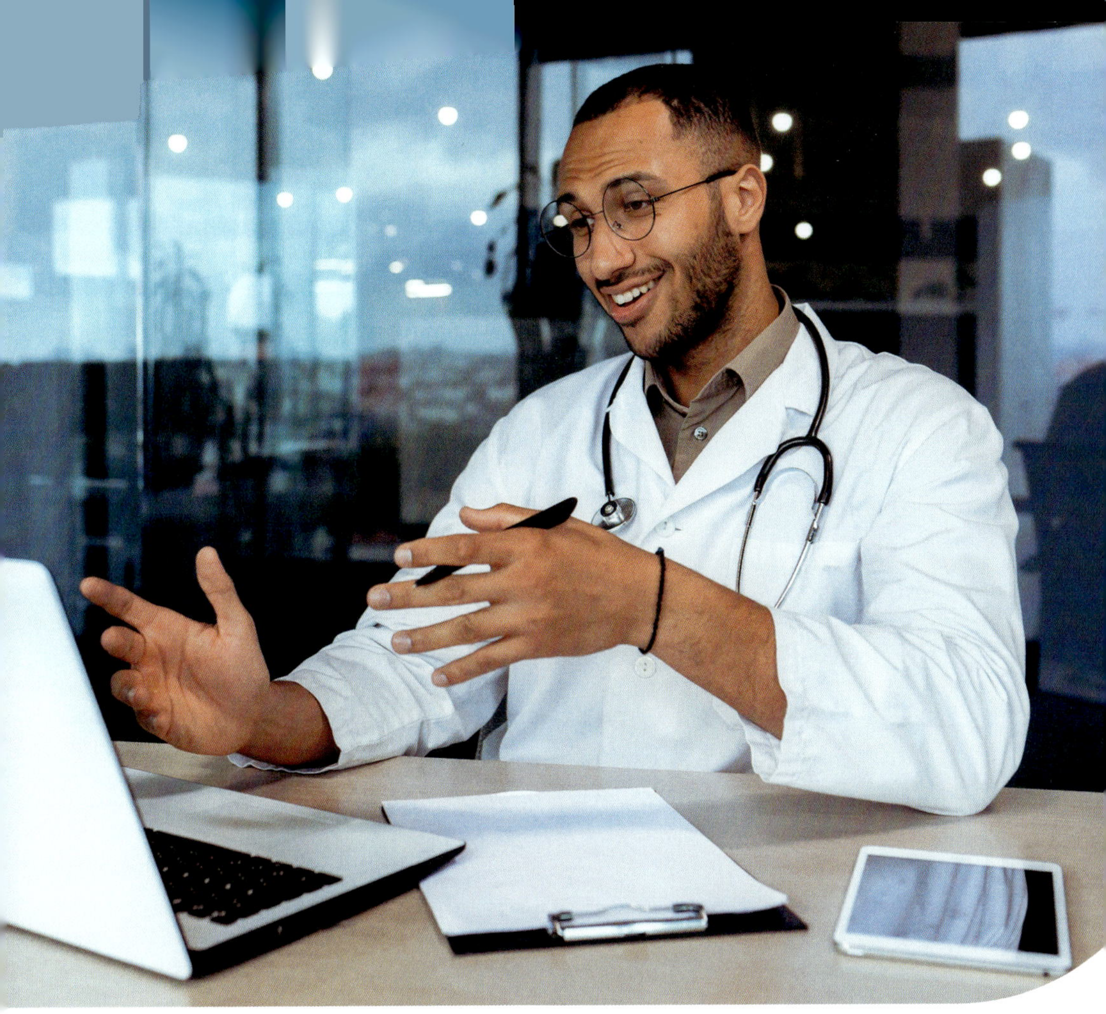

**Telehealth provides patients with easier access to health care professionals.**

They gain additional skills and experience needed for a specific field of medicine. Each path has its own challenges and rewards. PAs have to work hard. But these opportunities can lead to a lifelong career. Karis Kellner is a PA and director of clinical education. She works at the University of Arizona PA program. She says,

> *PAs are positioned to play a crucial role in the future of health care through an expanding scope of practice, leadership opportunities, advancements in education and the integration of technology. The future looks bright!*[7]

## Other Careers for PAs

PAs have many career options. They may become teachers who train other PAs. Others may become coaches who help people live a healthier life. Health insurance companies hire PAs to help approve insurance claims. Some PAs become medical writers. Medical writers help write documents such as educational materials.

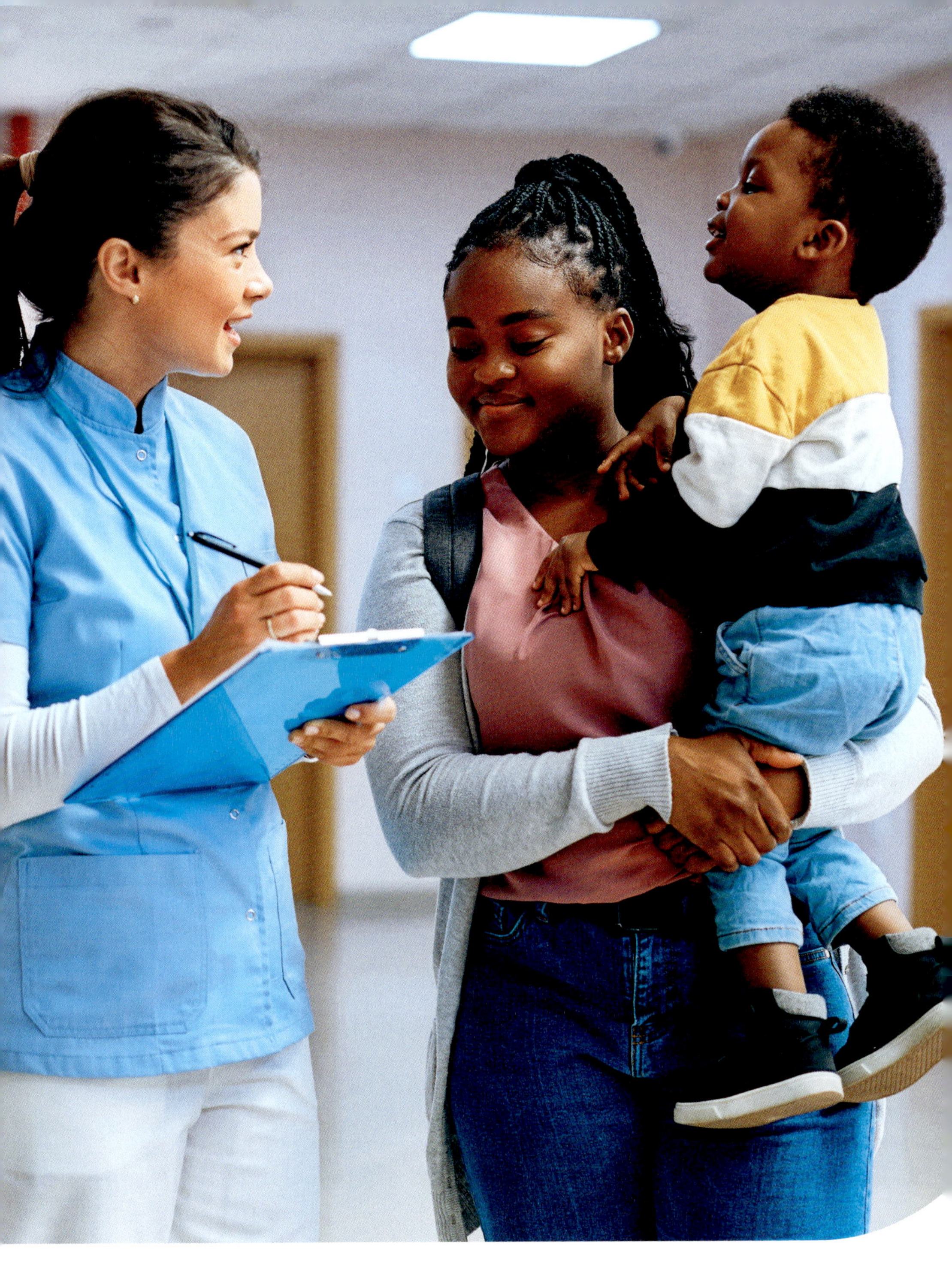

Health care staff make sure patients are taken care of during visits.

# GLOSSARY

**agencies**

parts of a government that oversee certain projects

**collaboration**

working together to accomplish a common goal

**diabetes**

a chronic disease in which the body has trouble controlling sugar levels in the blood

**elevated**

raised

**intensive care unit (ICU)**

a unit in a hospital or clinic where health care workers care for patients who are dangerously ill or injured

**rheumatology**

a medical field that treats diseases that affect the body's joints, muscles, tendons, and immune system.

**sanitize**

to make something clean and safe

**terminology**

special words used in a specific field of study or work

# SOURCE NOTES


## CHAPTER ONE: WHAT DOES A PHYSICIAN ASSISTANT DO?

1. Amber Davis, "PAs Advocate for Patients—And Improve the Health of Entire Communities," *PAs Go Beyond*, n.d. www.aapa.org.

2. "Physician Assistant," *Mayo Clinic*, n.d. https://college.mayo.edu.

3. Quoted in Vanessa Lane, "Becoming A Physician Assistant: Sadie's Story," *Concordia University Wisconsin*, October 13, 2021. https://blog.cuw.edu.

## CHAPTER TWO: BECOMING A PHYSICIAN ASSISTANT

4. Diana Anderson, "The Ups and Downs of My First Year as a PA," *American Academy of Physician Associates*, June 22, 2020. www.aapa.org.

## CHAPTER THREE: A DAY IN THE LIFE OF A PHYSICIAN ASSISTANT

5. "A Day in the Life of a Family Medicine Physician Assistant," *All Things PA*, July 14, 2020. https://allthingspac.com.

6. Adrijana Anderson, "A Day in the Life of a PA in Hospital Internal Medicine," *American Academy of Physician Associates*, August 14, 2022. www.aapa.org.

## CHAPTER FOUR: THE OUTLOOK FOR PHYSICIAN ASSISTANTS

7. Karis Kellner, "Five Emerging Trends in the Physician Assistant Profession," *University of Arizona Health Sciences*, October 8, 2024. https://healthsciences.arizona.edu.

# FOR FURTHER RESEARCH

## BOOKS

Kari Cornell, *Become a Diagnostic Medical Sonographer*. BrightPoint Press, 2025.

Margaret J. Goldstein, *Heroes of the Pandemic*. Lerner Publications, 2022.

Marne Ventura, *Be a Nurse Practitioner*. BrightPoint Press, 2026.

## INTERNET SOURCES

Adrijana Anderson, "A Day in the Life of a PA in Hospital Internal Medicine," *American Academy of Physician Associates*, August 14, 2022. www.aapa.org.

Victor Ouma, "Undergraduate Degrees for a Physician Assistant (With FAQs)," *Indeed*, October 7, 2024. www.indeed.com.

"The Physician Assistant Career: What Is a PA?" *Central Michigan University*, September 27, 2023. www.cmich.edu.

## WEBSITES

### American Academy of Physician Associates

**www.aapa.org**

The website of the American Academy of Physician Associates is a professional resource for PAs. They can learn about different aspects of the PA career and look for jobs in the field.

### Explore Health Careers

**https://explorehealthcareers.org**

The Explore Health Careers website takes a look at many different types of health care jobs and opportunities.

### Mayo Clinic: Explore Healthcare Careers

**https://college.mayo.edu**

The Mayo Clinic website provides an overview of the PA role. It includes information about what PAs do and what education and training are required.

# INDEX

# IMAGE CREDITS

Cover: © PeopleImages.com-Yuri A./Shutterstock Images
5: © Stock Photograph 3645/Shutterstock Images
7: © Ground Picture/Shutterstock Images
8: © R Photography Background/Shutterstock Images
9: © didesign021/Shutterstock Images
11: © PeopleImages.com-Yuri A./Shutterstock Images
13: © fizkes/Shutterstock Images
15: © fizkes/Shutterstock Images
16: © PeopleImages.com-Yuri A./Shutterstock Images
19: © Studio Romantic/Shutterstock Images
20: © PeopleImages.com-Yuri A./Shutterstock Images
22: © Gerain0812/Shutterstock Images
26: © Red Line Editorial
27: © Ken Wolter/Shutterstock Images
29: © tilialucida/Shutterstock Images
30: © PeopleImages.com-Yuri A./Shutterstock Images
33: © fizkes/Shutterstock Images
34: © pics five/Shutterstock Images
37: © Mangostar/Shutterstock Images
39: © Halfpoint/Shutterstock Images
41: © fizkes/Shutterstock Images
43: © SaiArLawKa2/Shutterstock Images
44: © Lysenko Andrii/Shutterstock Images
47: © Ground Picture/Shutterstock Images
49: © Monkey Business Images/Shutterstock Images
50: © PeopleImages.com-Yuri A./Shutterstock Images
53: © fizkes/Shutterstock Images
55: © voronaman/Shutterstock Images
57: © Drazen Zigic/Shutterstock Images

# ABOUT THE AUTHOR

Amy C. Rea grew up in northern Minnesota and now lives in a Minneapolis suburb with her family. She writes frequently about traveling around Minnesota and loves spending time with her family and her silly dog.